PHOTOGRAPHY
by NAZLI DEVELI

DESIGN
by STUDIO AURORA

EDITOR
STELLA NILSSON

All rights reserved. Copyright 2023 by Nazlı Develi
This book or any portion thereof may not be reproduced or used in any manner whatsoever without the express written permission of the publisher except for the use of brief quotations in a book review.

Hardcover Edition - First Printing, February 2023
ISBN 9798987853603
Independently published by Nazlı Develi

For information about permission to reproduce selections
from this book, write to hello@gurmevegan.com
www.gurmevegan.com
www.greenandawake.com

RAW FIKA

THE MOST LOVED SWEDISH PASTRY RECIPES
WITH A TOUCH OF BIG WIDE WORLD

"Raw Fika" is a modern dessert book for out-of-the-box thinkers who crave new ways to make fika treats that are honest, kind and delicious.

All recipes are raw, vegan, gluten-free.

RAW FIKA

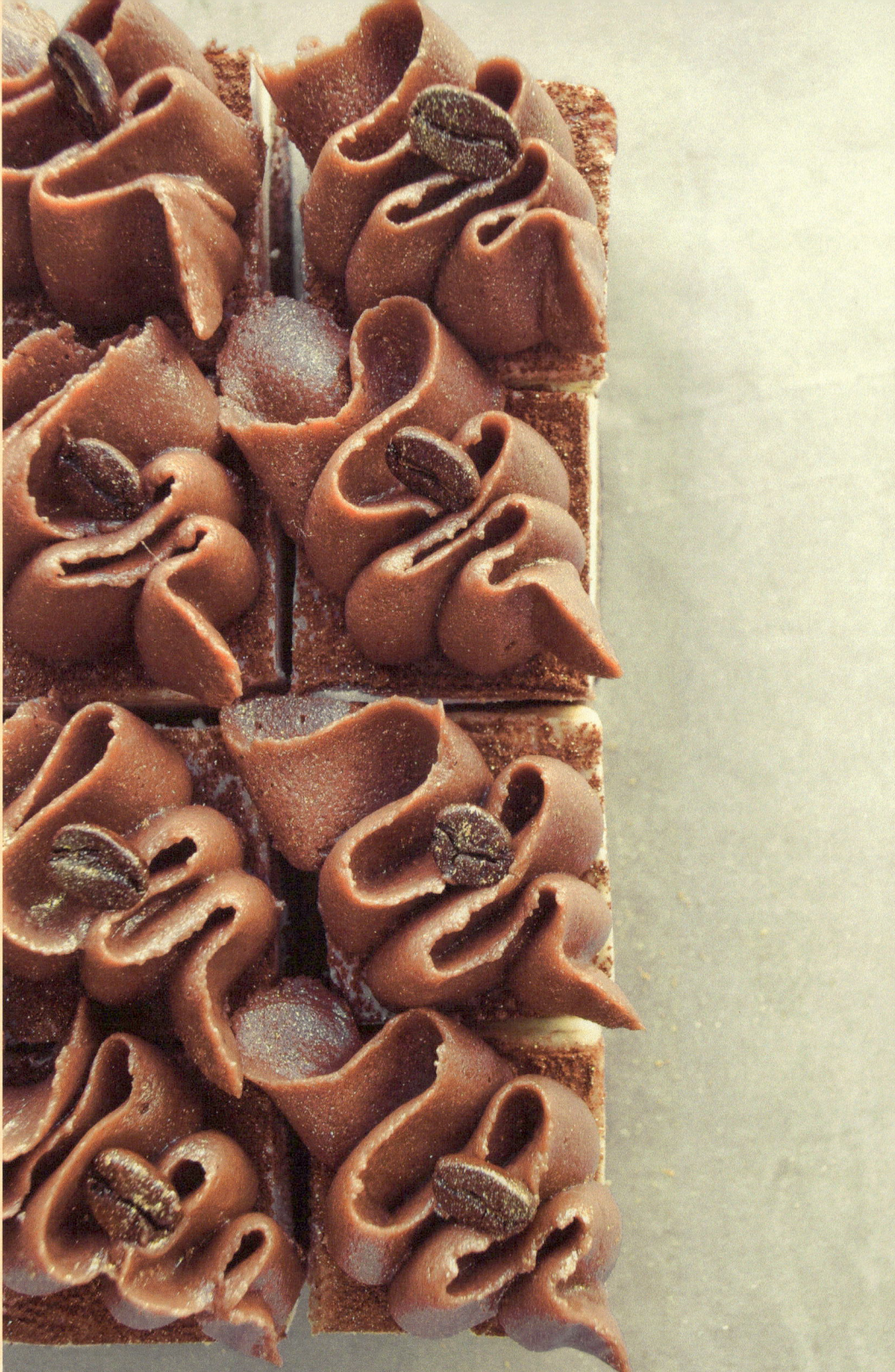

CONTENT

Introduction	6-7
Swedish Pastry Calendar	8-11
Before You Get Started	12
Fika Pantry Glossary	13-23
Equipments	24-25
Make-Ahead Fika Staples	26-31
Raw Fika Recipes	33-131
Index	132-134
About the Author	135

INTRODUCTION

Fika is a concept, a state of mind, an attitude and an important part of Swedish culture. Somewhat simpler and more spontaneous than the Brits' afternoon tea tradition.

Fika is both noun and verb and when in Sweden, it is essential to make time for fika every day. It means making time for yourself to reflect, or with friends and colleagues - and typically involves a cup of coffee and a sweet bite to eat. "Swedish cinnamon buns", "semla", "chocolate balls" or "vacuum cleaner" being arguably the most popular fika accompaniments.

But, of course, not everyone prefers coffee. To have a tea, cold press juice or any other drink instead is just as fine. You can also eat something savory instead of sweet. But Swedes don't tend to pair savory stuff with coffee: that honor goes to baked goods.

Loosely even if fika means a "coffee and sweet break" but that hardly captures the social significance of the term. Fika is the Swedish ritual of slowing down, creating a conscious space for yourself and finding beauty in moments, it's mostly social but also can be done alone. Some will say it's the very fabric of Swedishness.

Other Scandinavian countries have similar rituals around the coffee break, but they don't call it fika. In both Danish and Norwegian, the coffee break is called a "kaffepause."

The word fika actually derives from the 19th-century slang word for coffee, kaffi. It's pretty simple: Invert the word kaffi, and you get fika. kaffi -> ffi-ka -> fika

At many working places, fika is a part of the regular daily schedule. In the morning, a fika at 10:00 and in the afternoon at 15:00 is very common.
That means two 10 – 30 minutes extra breaks, called "fikarast" or "fikapaus".

During leisure time, fikas tend to be a little longer than working times. From 30 minutes to several hours. You can meet your friends, someone you have a common interest with and want to exchange ideas.

While Swedes love their traditional fika breaks, they are also health conscious and trend aware. It follows that Swedish food producers are among the world leaders of dairy-free, gluten-free and raw food alternatives.

The raw food trend is growing like crazy in Sweden. More and more cafés and restaurants are jumping on the healthy food and serving uncooked food and vibrant raw pastries, even in the small towns of Sweden. The choice of raw food includes everything from chia pudding and chocolate balls to innovative variations on classic dishes, nutrition-dense raw snacks and amazing raw cakes. Usually organic too, as well as refined sugar, gluten and dairy-free.

In this book, our fika recipes include some of the most popular Swedish buns, cakes, balls and cookies with a touch of big wide world. All raw, feel-good and perfect for your cozy fika moments. Each recipe creates its own ambiance and feeling that is attacted to food. You will find more detailed information in the recipes.
If you are new to raw food, you'll shortly realize that it actually can even be easier than the traditional baking.
On the other hand, raw dessert recipes developed today sometimes take a very long time, even days, as a dehydrator is used.
We are sure that most of you have limited time in your daily life for preperation of the recipe. That's why we included some of our recipes with two options: which you can mostly make by sitting them in the fridge, or dehydrating in a raw food dehydrator.

Although the use of a dehydrator is useful for long-term storage of some raw ingredients, it will never replace the actual nutritious raw food, as it also absorbs all the water content in the food and dries it. So if you don't have a dehydrator, don't worry and enjoy the most vibrant raw desserts.

This book is intended to inspire you to create your own healthy fika sweets that are "kind" without any harm to animals, "honest" which means healthy so there is nothing to hide in the ingredient list and "delicious" even more than traditional ones as raw is made with minimally processed, real ingredients.

Food Designer, Chef & Author

SWEDISH PASTRY CALENDAR

There are all kinds of Swedish goodies to satisfy everyone's tastes.

If you have a sweet tooth, you can't resist Swedish pastries because there are always excuses to have something sweet during all the day in Sweden. Take a look at the calendar below for special celebration days in Sweden.

January
In Sweden semla buns day (fettisdagen) is celebrated between Christmas and Easter. The bun, flavoured with cardamom and filled with almond paste and whipped cream. Semlor are available at bakeries every day from Christmas until Easter. We have three varieties of this delicious bun in the book.

There is also marzipan day (marsipanens dag) - a confection consisting primarily of sugar, sweetener, and almond meal, on January 12. You will find a chessboard cookies (schackrutor) recipe made of raw marzipan in this book.

Swedes also get a slice princess cake (prinsesstårta) since 12th of january is a Marzipan day. Prinsesstårta are mostly reserved for birthdays and other celebrations. You will also find our raw twist for prinsesstårta.

February
February 3 is the day of carrot cake (morotskakans dag). Our raw version in the book is a delicious take-on of traditional one, served with delicious sunflower cheesecake cream.

March
Then we come to March 7th, there is a special day for what we call "dammsugare" which means "vacuum cleaner" because their shape is reminiscent of a vintage cleaning appliance, or punch roll day (punschrullens dag), similar to the Danish træstammer and rumkugler that had been soaked in a spiced arrack-liqueur called Punsch. This pastry is easy to find in any confectionery and is traditionally colored green (sometimes yellow and pink) with chocolate coating in both ends. We have three varieties; yellow, bounty and traditional green version, made from scratch in the book. Yellow one and bounty style don't require arrack extract which might be hard to find for some who live outside Sweden.

March 25th is the official waffle day (våffledagen) in Sweden, Swedish waffles are a little bit different than famous Belgium waffles. They are thinner, usually made like a four-leaf clover where you get four hard shapes in one waffle. The most common way to eat them with fresh berries and whipped cream.

April

Licorice day (lakritsdagen) is celebrated on April 12 and every year a big lakrits fair is held in Stockholm. During this period of time you can see all things made with laktrits. Licorice comes in all shapes and sizes in Sweden. The most popular are soft gelatin candies.

Another most common way to consume licorice is to combine it with raspberry powder (hallon pulver) and cover it in chocolate. Salty licorice is also another popular combination in Sweden. It seems very bitter and impossible to eat to non-Swedish eyes. When in doubt, it is best to combine it with chocolate.

May

The 11th of May is chocolate ball day (chokladbollens dag). A Swedish classic which combines all the elements you'd ever need. They're creamy, chocolatey, rich, and is so easy to whip together they're one of the first things children learn to bake in Sweden. This sweet little balls are made with cacao and sugar of your choice and oats, and then rolled in either desiccated coconut or cacao.

May 15th is cardamom bun day (kardemummabulles dag) started to celebrate by some bakers who love this bun in Sweden. Cardamom buns are similar to cinnamon rolls except that they're smaller, knotted, and baked with lots of the aromatic spice.

In May, we also celebrate the muffins (muffindagen). I know muffins are really not a Swedish bakery product, but it is still appreciated and has its very own day in Sweden and that day is May 27. They are mostly made with blueberries freshly picked from the forest.

June

National Day has its very own tasty pastry called "nationaldagsbakelse" and celebrated on June 6. It is a naturally gluten-free marzipan crust cake, filled with almond and orange juice, topped with Swedish strawberries, which was chosen in a competition back in the 1990 and was created by Helena Bergsmark at Cafe Gateau in Stockholm.

During midsummer (the night before the longest day of the year) which takes place on a Friday between 19 and 25 June, there is also a special cake called midsummer cake (midsommartårta) or strawberry cake (jordgubbstårta) - a traditional Swedish strawberry layer cake enjoyed all throughout the strawberry season, there are many varieties of this cake but usually made with strawberries, vanilla cream and whipped cream. You will find our raw version with strawberry gel and coconut cream in the recipes section.

July

There's no cake or pastry to celebrate in July. But some people love baking sockerkaka (sponge cake).

August
Rolled cake day (rulltårtans dag) on August 9. Rulltårta comes in many forms and varieties but the two most common are the vanilla sponge with jam filling and the chocolate sponge with buttercream and berries inside. Even it is not swedish, it is very common in Sweden and we have a delicious reinterpreted version with black forest flavour.

Raspberry caves or Swedish raspberry thumbprint (hallongrottor) is also common this month. They're cute and delicate little bites of fruity and cookie heaven which in Sweden usually are filled with raspberry jam. Our version is made with soft zucchini dough, most people said that they are much more better than traditional one.

September
Oat crumble cake with apple and vanilla sauce (äppelsmulpaj) is usually made during September. Raw version is decadent take on of traditional one. They can be made by marinating as well as sous -vide cooking according to your preference.

The last week of September is the week dedicated for Swedish princess cake (prinsesstårta). You will find also learn how to make strawberry raw marzipan roses in the related recipe.

October
Sweden is considered its home of cinnamon bun (kanelbulle) . Cinnamon bun was created in the early-1900s but, as a result of war rations, was actually too expensive for most Swedes to eat.

So, cinnamon buns didn't enter the national psyche until the 1950s, when sugar prices went down and home baking went up.

Today, the cinnamon bun is the unofficial symbol of fika and is celebrated nationally on October 4th, cinnamon bun day (kanelbullens dag).
We have two version of kanelbulle, one is made with date caramel, and other one is with chocolate.

Gräddtårtans Dag (cream layer cake) on October 6.
You will find a gräddbulle recipe in the book.

November
Gustav Adolfsbakelse day (Gustav Adolf's cake) on November 6.

Swedish mud cake (kladdkakans dag) is a chocolate cake covered with sugar, berries and whipped cream. It lies somewhere between a brownie and a gooey lava cake. It is celebrated on November 7.

Our raw version of kladdkaka is very simple to make; the crust is similar to chokladbollar with a quick chocolate ganache, served with heavenly chunky monkey ice cream which is became very popular in Sweden these days.

Chokladens Dag (chocolate day) on November 11. You can make any kind of chocolate cake you like on this day.

Cheesecake day (Ostkakans Dag) falls on November 14. It is the Swedish version of a cheesecake called ostkaka, served at room temperature with berry jam and cream. Any kind of raw cheseecake is just fine. We recommend our Swedish blueberry cake for this day.

Wienerbrödets Dag (Wiener bread day) on November 22.

December
Across the Nordics, Advent Sunday marks the beginning of the Christmas season and continues the fourth Sunday before Christmas, and Swedes use first advent day to decorate their home, light the first of four candles in the advent wreath (adventsljusstake), drink mulled wine (glögg) and eat gingerbread cookies or balls (pepparkakor or pepparkaksbollar)

There is also a day for gingerbread cookies (pepparkakans dag) on December 9. You will find most nutritious gingerbread balls (pepparkaksbollar) recipe in the book.

Kakans dag (cake day – can be eaten any cake) on December 18.

In mid-December, on the shortest day in the medieval Julian calendar, Swedes get up early to celebrate Saint Lucy's Day (Luciadag). St. Lucia Buns (lussekatter) are made on December 13.

Lussekatter can be made raw or dehydrator baked according to your choice.
Swedish Christmas is celebrated on Christmas Eve (December 24th) over a christmas table (julebord).

Lastly, no Swedish Christmas meal would be complete with a rice porridge (risgrynsgröt) slow-cooked with milk and cinnamon. One almond is hidden in the entire pot, and it is believed that whomever finds it will get married in the coming year.

We have a raw version of rice porridge which is made with riced kohlrabi, raisins, almond butter and christmas spices. It is a vibrant and nutritious recipe that we highly recommend to try.

BEFORE YOU GET STARTED

The chapter provides an easy-to-read introduction to basic rules of raw food that you need to know while making our recipes.

WHAT IS RAW FOOD?

A food is considered raw if it has never been heated over 46°C.

Foods dehydrated at higher temperatures are not considered completely raw, but very lightly cooked as the moisture is removed. Cooking denatures many of these nutrients including delicate enzymes, vitamins, minerals and amino acids, affecting the nutrition of the product.

Keep in mind that dehydrated raw foods may take up to one-third longer drying times than called for in typical dehydration recipes, depending on climate, dehydrator type and liquid amount of the veggies or product.

Raw food should also not be refined, pasteurized, treated with pesticides or otherwise processed in any way. Beside dehydration, raw food diet allows several alternative preparation methods, such as juicing, blending, dehydrating, soaking, marinating and sprouting.

Similar to veganism, the raw food diet is usually plant-based. Some raw foodists also use bee pollen or honey. We never use animal based ingredient in our recipes. So we can describe our kitchen as raw vegan.

Time

All recipes in this book have rough time estimates. Because the actual time varies from person to person depending on your experience and the equipments you have.
But I do believe the estimate time will give you an indication of whether it takes too long or short.

Measurements

A digital kitchen scale is a must when making our recipes in this book. Weighing will give you consistent results every time. When you weighed 1 cup coconut flour using different volume measuring cups, as a test, you will notice every single one gives a different amount of grams. So it is best to use a scaler.

The Taste

Vegetables, fruits, nuts vary in size, variety, flavour, texture depending on season, ripeness, where and in which soil they have been growing.
Even I have covered my recipes detailed in the instruction parts, they may not be same dish in your kitchen. I tried to make the recipes easy and instructive as much as possible, but I kindly do ask that you taste recipes before you serve them, season according to your taste, check the texture, thickness and creamness.

FIKA PANTRY GLOSSARY

SWEDISH ITEMS

Lingonberry
A berry that you can associate with Sweden. It is picked in the wild woods in the end of August, beginning of September in Sweden. It has sour, bitter and a little rough in your mouth and tastes so good!
If you don't have access to lingonberries where you live in, you can use redberries, raspberries, sour cherries or your favorite type of berries. They are used in raw cakes both fresh and in powder form.

Licorice Salt
We use licorice salt in some of our recipes. It actually has no a strong flavour like licorice root. With notes of toasty nuttiness and a tangy licorice flavor licorice salt is a little salty, a little sweet, and all around delicious. It adds dimension to raw desserts. I highly recommend to get Icelandic licorice salt from Saltverk brand. It is possible to find this salt on Amazon as well. If you are not able to source, you can use pink himalayan salt.

Licorice Root Powder
In addition to being some of the top coffee drinkers worldwide, Swedes are also some of the highest consumers of candies per capita, particularly the salty varieties of licorice, which are flavored by salmiak, a salty powder.
It's a both bitter and sweet, just what Swedes need in the dark and long winters. They need licorice to get their blood pressure up and heat in their bodies.

There are many varieties of licorice. Compared to licorice extract powder, this licorice root powder contains only dried and ground licorice root, it's lighter in colour and the fibers are visible. We'd recommend Urtekram's licorice root powder to use in raw desserts. It is a Danish brand, common in Europe but can be found online or you can look for alternatives in your country.

Licorice root also has a wide range of health benefits, not only for digestion but also for skin, respiratory and urinary tract health. Licorice root also promotes immune function and has antioxidant properties. It also supports muscle and bone health and energy levels. However, if you suffer from high blood pressure, then you should avoid licorice...

Arrak/ Arrack Extract / Swedish Punsch Aroma
Arrak originally comes from Asia and it is a very strong aniseed spirits based on rice and molasses, very popular to use in Swedish chocolate balls and dammsugare. The sweet-sour taste and the strong smell make Arrak a perfect flavor for both pastries and drinks such as Punsch.
If you are living outside of Sweden, you can try sourcing it online through Amazon. We also have alternative recipes which don't require arrak in this book.

CACAO PRODUCTS

Raw Cacao Powder
Cocoa powder and cacao powder are very similar, the only difference being that cocoa is processed at a much higher temperature (and often packaged cocoa contains added sugar and dairy). Both start out as beans from the cacao plant, which are separated from the fatty part known as cocoa butter. We use raw cacao which is not exposed to high heat, in raw food desserts. Raw cacao powder is full of nutritious when compared with cocoa powder. If you are new to raw cacao, you might find unprocessed cacao powder is actually a bit bitter. Its strong taste is a result of the powerful nutrients that are present in unprocessed cacao, particularly its unique antioxidants. It's a seriously hardcore dark chocolate, and your body will thank you for it.

Raw Cacao Mass
Cacao mass or chocolate liquor is raw unsweetened chocolate produced from the whole pure cacao beans, liquified then cooled in a semi-solid or solid form.
We mostly use cacao mass with cacao butter and maple or coconut sugar in raw dessert recipes. You can make your own beforehand or use a high quality packaged raw chocolate to use in the recipes which require raw chocolate.
Raw cacao mass also makes for a great ingredient for flavouring ice cream, ganaches, pralines or other ingredient bases to achieve a deeper, darker colour and more intense cacao taste.

Raw Cacao Nibs
Raw cacao nibs are small pieces of crushed cacao beans that have a bitter, chocolatey flavor. We use them in balls, cookies (instead chocolate chips) and cake crusts.

BUTTERS AND OILS

Raw Cacao Butter
Raw cacao butter is a type of fat that comes from cacao beans, known as a mood boosting which can even help lower blood cholesterol levels. Cocoa butter has a mildly sweet flavor and aroma that is reminiscent of chocolate; the scent is stronger than the taste. It is used as a binder in raw dessert recipes. Just like virgin coconut oil, but cacao butter has ability to solidify the texture more than coconut oil. It also can be used in the recipes when you need white chocolate flavour.

When a recipe calls melted raw cacao butter in this book, measure the butter then melt using bain marie method. Do not melt more than you need. Although it solidifies later, it spoils the structure and taste of this material over time.

Virgin Coconut Oil

Unrefined virgin coconut oil is oil that has been pressed from coconut meat and undergone no further processing, it makes a fantastic replacement for butter in raw cake recipes. When a recipe calls melted virgin coconut oil, the best way to melt coconut oil is to do this naturally.

You only need temperatures of 24° C to liquify your oil and less if you just need it to be a soft, creamy consistency. If the season's temperatures or the climate that you live in allow for it, this is the least invasive and healthiest way to melt coconut oil. Scoop out the amount of coconut oil that you need and put it in a bowl or in a jar. Leave it somewhere where it's warm. If it's in direct sunlight, which is ok for a little while, cover the jar with a cloth or piece of fabric.

If you are living in a cold climate, the best way is to melt coconut oil is in a hot water bath. This method is also known as "au bain marie".

You put the coconut oil in a bowl placed in a pan with simmering water, with the fire off, while stirring. The coconut oil will melt by itself from the temperature of the water.

If you're in a hurry and need to speed up the process, you can put the pan on a low heat. A similar method which is just a little bit more user-friendly is a double boiler. This is a pan existing of two pans that are on top of each other. The bottom pan is for the hot water and the top pan holds the food.

This method is very practical if you have a large amount of coconut oil to melt or other ingredients to add.

Raw Coconut Butter

Coconut butter is simply shredded coconut turned into creamy coconut butter. It tastes like straight coconut. It's lightly sweet and nutty.

The only difference is that when it's cold, it doesn't stay fluid enough like other nut butters, and it can solidify completely. You may need to use it by melting with bain marie.

Sesame Oil

A popular cooking oil used in Chinese, Japanese, and Middle Eastern cuisines, sesame oil is made from raw or toasted sesame seeds. We mostly use it in dehydrated dough recipes, it helps to emulsify the flours, veggies and binders. When buying, make sure it is made of raw sesame seeds and doesn't contain any other ingredient inside.

Extra Virgin Olive Oil

Extra virgin olive oil has a lower smoke point than regular olive oil, has the lowest acidity level of all olive oils, contains the most anti-oxidants of all olive oils, and has a lower percentage of oleic acid (monounsaturated fat). We use it in dehydrated cookie recipes.

MOST COMMON USED DEHYDRATED ITEMS

Activated Dehydrated Nuts

Most raw nuts, seeds and grains contain phytic acid in order to protect them in early stages of growth. Almonds, walnuts, and Brazil nuts have the highest amounts of phytic acid which can decrease the absorption of iron, zinc, magnesium, and calcium in human body. Almonds contain 9.4% phytic acid, walnuts contain 6.7% phytic acid, and Brazil nuts contain 6.3% phytic acid.

Unrefined grains have the highest amount of phytic acid because they contain the entire grain; the husk, bran. In raw food terms, in order to destroy major part of phytic acid, we soak nuts and seeds in water for 5-6 hours or overnight depending on the nut variety, and then dehydrate in the food processor.

When you soak whole grains, nuts and seeds in warm water overnight, you activate the enzyme phytase. This enzyme then works to break down phytic acid, which binds minerals like iron, calcium, and zinc. As phytase does its magic, it releases minerals in whole grains and makes them easier for your body to absorb.

Sprouted Whole Oats or Rolled Oats

Soaked, sprouted, dehydrated and then grinded whole oats. You can make your own as well as you can use store-bought one. We use this ingredient in cake crusts. It is a great flour that gives the dough crispness and satiety.

It is more appropriate to use sprouted whole oats flour in raw cake recipes. However, if you don't have time to make from scratch or can't find store-bought, no worries, rolled oats also work.
It is said that sprouting increases the protein6 and free amino acids in oats. Although lower in phytates to begin with, sprouting oats for 24 hours breaks down antinutrient phytates to improve the bioavailabilty of vitamins and nutrients. In addition, sprouted oats are higher in magnesium11 and GABA12 than raw oats.

To make your own, soak the oat groats in water for 12 hours. Rinse them well. Then put the groats in a sprouting device and place in a cool, dark location. Once the groats have sprouted, you can move them out of the dark. Give the groats one final rinse and then transfer to your dehydrator sheet, dehydrate at 46°C until fully dried. Once dehydrated you can now grind them in grain mill or a high speed blender into flour.

Buckini
One of the most common used grain in our recipes is activated dehydrated buckwheats. When a recipe calls buckini (activated dehydrated buckwheats), just soak buckwheats in water for 3-4 hours (if you are in a hurry you can also soak in warm water for 40 minutes), then rinse, spread on dehydrator sheet, dehydrate for 3-4 hours or until completely dried at 46°C, You can prepare in batches, store in a mason jar and use in your recipes.

You may also want to sprout buckwheats and then dehydrate to Increase nutrient availability. While soaking can break down the anti-nutrients that can block nutrient absorption, sprouting can increase the nutrient availability of a food. Several studies show that sprouting grains has increased their essential amino acids and other important vitamins. To sprout buckwheats, fill with lukewarm water in a 2 part water to 1 part buckwheat ratio. Allow it to soak for 1 hour at room temperature. The buckwheat will plump up and the water will most likely be a bright pinkish-red. Rinse them off and leave them at room temperature for 2 to 3 days. Continue to rinse them once or twice daily during that 2 to 3 days. Use the sprouted buckwheat immediately in your salads or dehydrate in the food dehydrator for 3-4 hours or until completely dried. Once they are dehydrated, you can name them buckini now, they will be ready to use in the raw cake crusts.

The other most common ingredient you will find in the recipes are cashews. We mostly use them for making cream, cheesecake filling. First we soak cashews in warm water for 2-3 hours, then rinse twice before using.
Sometimes we also use cashews in crusts, especially when we want the crust in light color. Then we need to soak cashews for 2 hours, rinse and then dehydrate at 46°C until completely dried.

While almonds need to be soaked for 8 hours and walnuts and pecans for 4 hours to activate, some nuts such as brazil nuts, macadamia and hazelnuts doesn't need to be soaked.

Chia Seeds

Chia seeds are an excellent source of fiber, which can improve heart health, reduce cholesterol levels and promote intestinal health. Fiber takes longer to digest and makes you feel satisfied longer. We use chia seeds in raw dessert crusts for more nutritional value and sometimes as a binding agent.

Psyllium Husk Powder

Psyllium is a form of fiber made from the husks of the Plantago ovata plant's seeds. It can help relieve both constipation and diarrhea, and is used to treat irritable bowel syndrome and other intestinal problems. Psyllium husk is the crucial ingredient in raw baking. It acts as a binder, and it gives the elasticity, flexibility and extensibility to dough it needs so you can actually knead and shape it easily.
When buying, make sure you get it in powder form.

Flaxseeds

Flaxseeds are a good source of dietary fiber and omega-3 fatty acids, including alpha-linolenic acid. We use flaxseeds for nutrition value or sometimes as a binder, similar to chia.
Chia seeds have slightly fewer calories and more fiber. They also have 2.5 times more of the bone-strengthening mineral calcium, as well as slightly more iron and phosphorus. Both seeds are very nutritious. If you're looking for more omega-3s, pick flax seeds.
You may need to grind the seeds in a spice grinder or mortar before using depending on the recipe. Grind only what you need to relish the freshness.

Hemp Seeds

Similar to chia or flax seeds, hemp hearts are jam-packed with nutrients, they are one of our pantry staples. Derived from the Cannabis Sativa plant, hemp hearts are simply the soft inner part of hemp seeds once they have been unshelled – their squishy centre, if you will. Despite sharing the same plant mother, hemp hearts don't contain CBD or THC, therefore will not make you feel high, just in case you were worried. They has nutty flavour and chewy texture. You can use them in raw cake dough, roll your bliss balls in hemp hearts or add some in cashew cream while making fillings, dosing up on hemp hearts is one of many plant-based ways we can increase our protein intake.

Maca Powder

Maca is derived from the root of a cruciferous vegetable native to Peru, and is related to broccoli, cauliflower and kale. The root, which is the edible part of the vegetable, looks similar to a cross between a parsnip and radish, with green, leafy tops. It's typically consumed as a ground powder.
It packs high levels of iron and iodine to promote healthy cells and to help keep your metabolism on track. Its big doses of potassium help digestion and make muscles happy. Maca is also rich in calcium. It tastes better when combined with cacao powder or carob powder. You can use it both in crusts and creams.

MOST COMMON USED INGREDIENTS FOR FILLINGS

Cashew

When it comes to raw desserts and icecream, cashews are something of a miracle ingredient. Their creamy taste and texture make them the perfect substitute for dairy without losing the flavour profile associated with a dairy ice cream.

When buying them, just make sure they are fair trade, organic and unroasted. Fair trade is so important because in some countries where cashews are peeled, women have to separate the actual nut from the skin, which contains toxic oils that burn skin and damage the eyesight. They are usually not provided with safety equipment such as gloves due to cost-cutting measures, which expose them to these toxins and influence their health and well-being.

Child labour is also common in the industry. According to the International Labour Organization, approximately 168 million children are forced to pick and deshell cashews.

Pine Nut

Alternatively you can also use pine nuts which are pretty sustainable, and cause no harm to land, soil, air, water and animals as long as no pesticides are used. Pine nuts resemble cashews in color, texture and mild sweetness, and can be used as a substitute in just about any recipe. Stick to unsalted raw versions for raw desserts.

Macadamia

When eaten fresh off the tree, the texture of macadamia nut is creamy, almost like the inside of a fresh coconut. They must be dried for storage and shipping. If you find fresh one, you are really lucky. They have unique texture and flavour. Even when dried, they still end up with a rich, buttery flavour. Similar to cashews, just a bit more buttery than cashews.

Young Coconut Meat

Young coconut meat harvested directly from the tree before it has time to age, it is a soft flesh edible part on the inside of a green coconut. This meat varies in texture and color, from a white gelatin-like material that is dense enough to be sliced to a nearly transparent, runny gel-like meat. It can be bought at some food stores in fresh or canned form.

We use young coconut meat instead cashews in white filling creams and frostings. It tastes so good and best alternative for those who have nut-allergy.

SWEETENERS

Coconut Nectar Syrup

Coconut nectar is the delicious syrup derived from the sap of the flowers of the coconut palm. When dehydrated into granules it becomes coconut sugar, but as a liquid, it's comparable to maple syrup or agave. We mostly choose coconut nectar to sweeten our raw desserts because it is natural and minimally processed.

Coconut nectar syrup is also a wonderful low GI sweetener, making it a superior alternative to maple syrup's high glycemic index.

Pure Maple Syrup

Maple syrup is made by concentrating the slightly sweet sap of the sugar maple tree, a healthier alternative to table sugar and a natural vegan alternative to honey and has many benefits. It's less processed than regular table sugars and therefore contains more nutrients like vitamins, minerals & antioxidants which help improve your health. As a liquid sweetener we prefer using maple or coconut nectar in our recipes.

If you are looking for a cheaper option, grape or mulberry molasses will still work althought they are not raw but there are some cold pressed fruit extracts such as grape, carob, mulberry that are close to raw.

Just make sure to use only in dark creams as it will change the color of white fillings.

Light Agave

Sometimes we also use light agave syrup even we don't prefer all the time as it has the highest fructose content of any commercial sweetener on the market. While some people are actively avoiding high fructose corn syrup with a fructose content of only 55%, they continue to receive agave due to its low glycemic index while without knowing consuming a product with 90% fructose. If you're using agave, it is best to use minimum amounts as much as possible.

Maple syrup has a distinct, full-bodied flavor, while agave syrup has a relatively neutral flavor. So this makes agave great sweetener in white buttercreams, both in terms of flavour and color.

Powdered Coconut Sugar

Coconut sugar (also known as coco sugar, coconut palm sugar, coco sap sugar or coconut blossom sugar) is a coconut palm sugar produced from the sap of the flower bud stem of the coconut palm.

It is often confused with palm sugar, which is similar but made from a different type of palm tree. A natural sweetener similar to brown sugar we use a lot in raw dessert recipes. Before you use them in recipes, grind in coffee or spice miller. Otherwise, it may sound irritating to your mouth in the form of crystal granules.

Erythritol and Monk Fruit Sweetener
Erythritol occurs naturally in a variety of foods (e.g., grapes, mushrooms, pears and watermelon) and some fermented foods and beverages like beer, cheese, sake, soy sauce and wine. But in powder form is also commercially produced using fermentation.
Erythritol is certainly the more attractive option for sufferers of fructose intolerance, since these molecules are even smaller than both sorbitol and xylitol. Although it is man-made and we do not fully embrace it in our kitchen, I can say that it is useful because we need a powdered sweetener as an alternative to white sugar in some recipes. After all, it's better than table sugar. Whether you use it or not is entirely up to you. Stevia and Xylitol are other alternatives that we do not prefer to use.
It usually can be used in raw dough recipes where you don't want dark color. When buying make sure that it is in powder form or you can grind it in coffee or spice mill into flour.
Another alternative can be monk fruit sweetener, it is a fruit with juice that's about 200 times as sweet as sugar and has zero calories. Monk fruit sweeteners are produced by removing the seeds and skin of the fruit, crushing the fruit, and then filtering and extracting its sweet portions into liquid and powdered forms, and considered as a natural sweetener.

Dates
Native to Morocco, Medjool dates are just one of hundreds of varieties of dates, but they're the only one known as "the fruit of kings." With a sweet, caramel taste and chewy texture, Medjool dates were originally eaten by royalty and thought to fend off fatigue. We use medjool variety a lot in raw desserts. When a recipe calls medjool dates in our recipes, it is given in grams in the ingredient list, this means they are weight after pitted. So make sure you removed the seeds of your dates, then measure before using. They can be used both in cake crusts and fillings as a caramel.

Raisins
Dried raisins have a moderately low glycemic index, which means they don't cause sharp spikes and dips in your blood sugar levels. This can make raisins a great sweet option for people with diabetes. You can use raisins instead dates for a cheaper option, or for a more distinct flavour.
In addition, dried fruits such as plums, apricots, gojiberries, mangoes and figs can be used as an alternative option.

FLAVOURS AND EXTRACTS

Vanilla Bean Powder or Extract

Vanilla powder is a fine powder made from dried, ground, and processed vanilla beans. Some products may also contain dextrose or cornstarch to keep the powder from clumping. So make sure you are buying from trusted source or use from whole vanilla beans.

You can also use homemade or store-bought vanilla extract. Homemade vanilla is more cost efficient than store-bought options. To make it yourself cut three vanilla beans open lengthwise for every cup of glycerin you use. Add the beans to the glycerin, making sure they're completely submerged. Then cap the bottle and store it in a cool, dark place. Shake the bottle once a week. For optimal flavor, wait at least 6-12 months before using.

Essential Oils

Essential oils can be used safely in cooking, but it's important to understand which oils are okay to use, which you should avoid and how much is considered safe. When buying, make sure that it is food grade. Most common essential oils we use in our desserts are orange, bergamot, lavender, rosemary, lemon, vanilla, coconut and peppermint. DoTERRA is most common essential oil brand used in raw desserts.

Extracts

The best way of adding brilliant, crisp flavour to your desserts is by using extracts such as coconut, chocolate, cherry. Medicine Flower Flavour Extracts are most common brand used in raw desserts. If you find another brand in your country and trust the source, you can use it as well.

Sunflower Lecithin Powder

Sunflower Lecithin is an emulsifying agent that helps fat and liquid stay together. It is often added to foods such as chocolates, creams, icecreams, dressings.

It is is rich in choline, an essential nutrient similar to B vitamins. It regulates vital bodily functions including promoting a healthy nervous system. Choline is often converted into acetylcholine, a neurotransmitter that plays a role in learning, memory, and other aspects of the brain.

When buying it, make sure that it is in powder form. It is not a must ingredient in raw cakes but when you add a teaspoon to your fillings which especially contain more liquid, you will notice the difference.

NATURAL COLOURINGS WE LOVE THE MOST

Butterfly Pea Flower (Blue)
Butterfly pea powder is made from the butterfly pea plant, a beautiful flowering vine native to Thailand, Burma and other parts of Southeast Asia. It's bright indigo flowers have been used for centuries to dye foods various shades of blue.

Red Pitaya, Hibiscus & Beetroot Powder (Red and Pink)
They are used to dye foods various shades of pink and red. Just experiment in different amounts to see which tone is best for you.

Turmeric Powder & Gojiberries (Yellow & Orange)
When you make a mango cake, you will notice that it doesn't have enough color in it, then a pinch of turmeric would help. Another great ingredient you can get yellow and slightly orange color from it, is gojiberries. Just soak some gojiberries in warm water then use together with its water in raw cakes.

Japanese matcha Powder (Light Green)
Matcha is a powder that's made of finely ground green tea leaves from the Camellia sinensis plant which can be used for coloring in raw desserts. Quality matcha should be bright green; electric green.
Bad matcha will be a dull green; some are even army green, others are downright yellowish. These colors are bad qualilty sign of matcha.

Spirulina (Dark Green)
Spirulina is often classified as a superfood due to its extremely high content of nutrients, prepared from the biomass of blue-green algae. Spirulina is natually dark green in color, while Blue Majik has a vibrant cyan blue color.

Thai pandan Powder (Emerald Green)
Pandanus amaryllifolius or pandan is widely used as a source of natural seasoning such as food coloring and flavoring. Pandan can be used as a substitute for vanilla whenever a recipe calls for it to add another dimension of flavor to a dessert. We recently discovered this unique item during our visit to Asia. It also can be ordered online on Amazon. We add pandan to our desserts for nuanced flavor and a subtle green hue.

EQUIPMENTS

Food Processor
From the simplest to the most professional, the product in your hand will probably meet your needs when making raw dough. The food processor is of little importance, as there is no need for a smooth consistency like cream in base doughs. If you have a good blender, it is easy to grind the nuts, seeds and grains into flour first and then put them in the food processor. If you're looking for purchasing new one, we would recommend Cuisine Art.

Blender
The blender is one of the essential kitchen tools you need to make smooth raw creams. If you own a Blendtec with wide-side and twister jar, or an equally good quality blender, your work will be much easier. A blender can't quite replace all of the features of a food processor like the grating blade, so you will need both a blender and food processor.
I do not recommend this product completely even though I am satisfied with its performance after I have used for years, by the time I became very uncomfortable by its noise and vibration due to its high power. Decide by doing your own research.

Food Dehydrator
Dehydrators are widely used in raw cuisine, also very cost-effective in the long-run. They allow you to buy produce in bulk, especially when it is in season or on sale, and store it to use later on. They're also a great tool for gardeners who often have a surplus of ingredients on hand.
Although food dehydrators are useful in enabling food for storage, running it everyday and dehydrating everything for long hours even days may not make much sense. As with everything, it has advantages and disadvantages. It is a product that will be very beneficial as long as it is used in balance.
If you don't have a dehydrator, don't worry, because it is much better to consume the minerals and water without drying the food.
It is wonderful for storing nuts and grains by dehydrating them after soaking process, great for creating crispy elements and decorating your cakes. Ideal for making some gourmet cookies and pie bases and raw jams, also for thawing frozen creams at low temperature.
Today, unfortunately, most people still have microwaves in their homes that expose them to excessive radiation. If you can, it's much better to have a dehydrator at home instead of the microwave.

Coffee or Spice Grinder
Coffee or spice grinders are a lot quicker to use than a traditional mortar and pestle. All you have to do is put the spices in, hold down the button, until it's grounded up to your liking. You can do cinnamon sticks, cloves, star anise, cinnamon, chia, flaxseeds, coconut sugar and so many more.

Cake Molds

We generally work with 15 cm moulds in our recipes.

15x15 cm square mold: You will get 9 or 12 square cakes depending on your cut size, or 6-9 long cake bars when cut lengthwise.

15 cm round cake mold: You can serve the 15 cm round cake by dividing it into 6 equal parts.

5-7cm cake rings: It is also recommended to have 5 and 7 cm cake molds for miniature-like cakes, nested cakes.

Double Boiler

Double boilers are two pots that use steam as a heat source to melt something. They are made up of two pieces, a large pot that is filled with hot or boiling water and a smaller pot that fits inside and uses the steam from the hot water to heat your butter. You will need it to melt cacao butter and coconut oil.

Thermometer

While melting with a double boiler, keep the stove as low as possible and it may be useful to check it with a thermometer so that it does not increase above 46°C. The thermometer is necessary if you are going to make raw chocolate from scratch.

Measuring Spoons

Measuring spoons are special, standardized spoons used to measure very small quantities of ingredients by volume quickly and accurately. The ingredients measured can be liquid, or dry. A standard, no-frills set of measuring spoons will include 1/8 tsp, 1/4 tsp, 1/2 tsp, 1 tsp (teaspoon), and 1 tbsp (tablespoon).

For completeness in the book, we usually measure our ingredients in grams, but we list the spices in teaspoons in the ingredient lists since they are difficult to measure.

Scaler

Using a scale is the only way to avoid discrepancies in your measures. It may seem time-consuming at first, but the end result is fewer dirty dishes, less mess, a better yield and more consistent results. Our recipe ingredients are given in grams. Make sure you have a scaler before getting started.

Pastry Bag & Piping Set

A pastry bag is a conical kitchen tool with a small hole at the very end, fit for cake decorating tips. You squeeze the pastry bag with your hands and apply a degree of pressure to create detailed patterns.

Ruler

Especially if you are making professional cakes or want your cuts to look even, you can cut them in equal pieces by marking with a ruler.

MAKE-AHEAD FIKA STAPLES

INGREDIENTS

Dark Chocolate Frosting
100 g cashews
22 g coconut sugar powdered
60 g coconut milk
50 g coconut cream
15 ml lemon juice
15 g raw cacao powder
75 g coconut oil melted
1/8 tsp pink himalayan salt

White Chocolate Frosting
100 g macadamia or cashews
40 g coconut milk
40 g coconut cream
50 g maple syrup
30 g coconut oil melted
20 g raw cacao butter melted
15 ml lemon juice
1/8 tsp pink himalayan salt

Coconut Frosting
150 g young coconut meat
100 g coconut cream
50 g coconut nectar syrup
30 g virgin coconut oil melted
20 g raw cacao butter melted
1 tsp sunflower lecithin powder
A pinch pink himalayan salt

INSTRUCTIONS

Dark Chocolate Frosting
Soak your cashews in lukewarm water for 4-5 hours. Then rinse, transfer to a high speed blender. Add powdered coconut sugar (grind the coconut sugar in coffee or spice mill beforehand). Then add coconut milk, coconut cream, lemon juice, raw cacao powder and pink himalayan salt. Blend until smooth. Lastly add melted coconut oil, process again until everything is well incomparated. Transfer frosting in an airtight container, freeze at least 5-6 hours or overnight. Remove from the freezer, sit in the room temperature for 1 hour or in the dehydrator at low temperature for 15 minutes before using for piping.

White Chocolate Frosting
Soak your cashews in lukewarm water for 4-5 hours. Then rinse, transfer to a high speed blender. Add coconut milk, coconut cream, maple syrup, lemon juice and pink himalayan salt. Blend until you get a silky smooth mixture. Lastly add melted coconut oil and cacao butter. Blend until well incomparated. Transfer frosting in an airtight container, freeze at least 5-6 hours or overnight. Remove from the freezer, sit in the room temperature for 1 hour or in the dehydrator at low temperature for 15 minutes before using for piping.

Coconut Frosting
Place young coconut meat, coconut cream, coconut nectar and salt into your blender. Blend until smooth. Then add melted coconut oil and cacao butter. Process again. Lastly add sunflower lecithin powder and blend until well incomparated. Since young coconut meat is more liquid in form than nuts, sunflower seed will provide a more consistent mixture here, so that the liquids are emulsified. Store in the freezer to solidify before piping.

Coconut Cream

There are many ways to make coconut cream. We love to make it from young coconut whenever possible. Alternatively, a good quality organic canned coconut milk is always one of our pantry staples. Options and tastes can vary, we always encourage experimentation and adjustment. Feel free to try the many options and do what feels, and tastes, best for you.

From young coconut meat
Before purchasing; note that young coconuts are green and most young coconuts have been shaved down before packing and shipping for easier use (the green outer husk is very difficult to get into!). They are harvested from the tree when young, before they mature into a hairy brown coconut, or sometimes they fall down by self.

It may be challenging to open a young coconut, there is many different ways to open it and it fully depends on both hardness of coconut and your skills with knifes. If you are not comfortable using knifes, in order not to take unnecessary risks with knifes, you may also use a hammer and a thin metal (like a nail, scewdriver etc.).

First you need to drain the coconut water in it. Shave the excess soft parts on the top. Find softest point (or dot if the coconut is more mature, brown / nearly brown), stick the thin metal there to make a hole, then drain the water into a cup.

To open the top/rest of the coconut, we should lead you to google some videos and see alternatives that is safer and fits better to your skills.

After it cracks open, use a butter knife or coconut spoon to separate the meat from the shell. Beware of the cracked sharp edges, may hurt your hands.
You can also make this process easier by using a tool called "coco jack" which is becoming famous in Sweden.

Once you have young coconut meat, put in a high speed blender, add some coconut water (just enough to add very little that the machine will spin). Process until you get smooth cream. Store in the mason jar and use within 2 days.

From shredded coconut
Combine one part water (or coconut milk, for a richer result) with four parts shredded unsweetened coconut (either fresh or dried desiccated) mix in a high speed blender.
Strain the mixture through cheesecloth, squeezing out as much of the liquid as possible. Keep in the refrigerator to solidify overnight.
Do not discard the pulp. Freeze the coconut pulp to use later in cake crusts or cookies.

From canned coconut milk
Chill 400 ml canned coconut milk in the refrigerator overnight. This will make the milk fat separate and solidify on top. Use a spoon to skim the solidified coconut cream from the top of the can and put it in a glass bowl. Reserve the remaining liquid for another use.
Liquid can be used in the recipes where coconut water is needed. You can now use solidified coconut cream in the recipes that call the coconut cream in this book.

Raw Chocolate Base

Some of our recipes in this book call for raw chocolate. You can either use a packaged raw chocolate you like the taste, or you can make it from scratch by following the recipe below.

Remember, making chocolate from scratch is a very long process and requires more practice to master. To make it easier, we've included one of the simplest below. If you're more interested in this topic, you can find more details in our "Gourmet Raw Cakebook".

Ingredients
300 g raw cacao mass
225 g raw cacao butter
175 g coconut nectar syrup
15 ml vanilla extract
1/8 tsp licorice salt

Instructions
Finely chop cacao paste and cacao butter using a chef knife. Place them in a large bowl. Dehydrate at 46°C for 45-50 hour until everything is melted.

Alternatively you can melt them using bain marie method. But then you will need a thermometer to check the temperature in the bowl in order not exceed 46°C.
Stir ocassionally to increase the speed of melting process.
Once melted, add the vanilla, coconut nectar and salt. Stir well until everything well combined.
If the mixture starts to thicken, place back in the dehydrator or bain marie.

Set your dehydrator to 31°C. Once all ingredients all combined, place the bowl in the dehydrator. Just wait for couple of minutes, check the chocolate in the bowl with a thermometer, once the temperature is 31°C, your chocolate is tempered.
Pour a drop on parchment paper, allow to cool. If it comes firm and shiny then it is correctly tempered. Now you can pour the chocolate in the mold you want. Let it cool and store. It is ready to use in your raw dessert recipes.

Avocado Chocolate Frosting

Avocado, known as the butter fruit in ancient times, allows you to get a more creamy texture without cashews. It's a great option, especially for those who have nut-allergy. We recommend that it be consumed within 3 days in the refrigerator. You can make it a day in advance before serving on the cake.

Ingredients
100 g ripe avocado meat
100 g coconut cream
70 g maple syrup
30 g raw cacao
40 g coconut oil melted
A pinch salt

Instructions.
Place peeled and cored ripe avocado meat in the food processor, add the coconut cream, maple syrup, raw cacao and salt. Process until smooth. Then add the melted coconut oil. Run your food processor again, mix everything until well incomparated. Taste it, add more maple or salt if you need. Refrigerate for few hours if you will pipe the cream on the cake. If it is too thick, just let it sit in the room temperature for couple of minutes before piping.

Fermented Cashew Cream

This is a fermented cashew base recipe for making raw cheesecakes. Instead soaking and throwing raw cashews to your blender, you can also ferment them beforehand to have far lighter and slightly sour flavour.

Ingredients
140 g cashews, soaked
60 ml water (just enough to blend)
2 capsules probiotic powder

Instructions
Soak your cashews, rinse and dry, add to a high speed blender, process with probiotic powder and just enough water to create a thick cream mixture. Pour the mixture into a glass jar, press cling film down on top of the mixture so as to not form a crust on top and place in a warm space for 12-24 hours.
The mixture should be aerated and slightly sour smelling when you check on it. Once cashews have fermented, give it a stir and then refrigerate for at least 4 hours to firm up. Now you can use it in raw desserts.

Raw Fruit Jams

There are two ways of making raw jams. One requires dehydrator while other one doesn't. You can choose which one is best for you. If you have time I highly recommend dehydrating it overnight, you will have a vibrant delicious raw jam in real jam texture in the morning.

Ingredients
250 g fruits of your choice
20 ml lemon juice
5 g chia seeds

From fresh fruits
Place fruits in a bowl, mash with a fork, add lemon juice, maple and chia seeds, mix well. Dehydrate at 42°C for 6 hours or until you get a thick fruit mixture.

Soak the dried fruits
Since dried fruit contains less water than fresh, you'll want to rehydrate it first.
Blend. Transfer the soaked fruit to a high-speed blender and blend on high until pureed.
Store. Leftover jam keeps well in an airtight container in the refrigerator for up to 1 month.

If your jam is too juicy, you may need to dehydrate longer. For a quick solution you can also add a half teaspoon (or more as needed) psyllium husk powder. Just make for couple of minutes to observe. Psyllium will absorb the water content from the mixture.
You can also add chia seeds, they work the same way. As long as you wait, they will absorb the water content from the jam.

Dehydrated Raw Cookie Base for Cake Crusts

Ingredients

8 g chia seeds + 60 ml filtered water
45 g sprouted oat flour
45 g almond flour
20 g raw cacao powder (add coconut flour instead, if you want blonde base)
10 g raw coconut sugar powdered
70 g coconut nectar syrup
60 g raw almond butter
40 g chopped raw chocolate (add 15 g melted cacao butter if you want blonde base)
10 ml extra virgin olive oil
2 g baking soda
A pinch pink himalayan salt

Instructions

In a mixing bowl, mix chia seeds and water. Keep stirring for the first minute or so to prevent the chia seeds from clumping together. Then set aside for 5 minutes.
Then add the rest of ingredients in the chia seed mixture. Stir well to combine.
Place the bowl in the freezer for 15 minutes. Once time is up, remove from the freezer. You will be able to work easier with the dough now. Roll it out between two pieces of teflex or greaseproof paper to about 1/4 inch thickness. Cut into squares and dehydrate at 42°C for 8 hours or overnight. You can make them beforehand and store in the airtight container. Just run into flour in the blender before using in raw cake crusts.

This is an advanced and delicious crust flour works great every time. Since I developed this recipe, I always have in my pantry and mostly use it in crusts instead only using nut flours.

Nut Butters

In raw food rules, nut butters are made without exposure to heat. However, if you like the taste of roasted nuts, you can blend them after roasting, depending on your choice. Some nuts are difficult to turn into butters such as hazelnuts, after the hazelnuts are lightly roasted and peeled, they release their oil and turn into nut butter easily.

To make nut butter cream, add nuts to high-speed blender or food processor blend until creamy, stopping frequently to scrape down the sides as needed. If adding in extra ingredients, please do so after you have achieved a creamy consistency.

The total time from beginning to end may take 10 to 25 min. depending on your machine. To make sure you get that super creamy texture, just when you think you're done. Keep the blender going for another 5 minutes or so.

Be sure if adding maple syrup it's a little warm (at room temperature preferred) before adding. If you add cold maple syrup your mixture will seize up a bit and take longer to finish.

Raw Date Caramel

Sukkari Dates which means 'the sweet one' has distinctive yellowish skin of acorn-shape and because of the crystallised sugars they contain can be slightly crunchy and also soft.

These golden dates are larger than Deglet Nour dates, with all the softness and caramel-like flavour of Medjools.
They are characteristically very sweet, and more succulent than standard dates. So we can say that sukkari dates are perfect to make date caramel.

Make sure you will use fresh dates for this. If your dates are dry, they won't blend as well and will require soaking in warm water first in order to soften them. Otherwise, you won't achieve that creamy, raw caramel-like consistency.
If you want a thicker consistency, reduce the water content in the recipe.

You do not need to peel off their skins, do not waste them, because their vitamins are right there! If you have a good blender and use slightly warm water, you will get a very nice consistency.

Ingredients
120 g fresh sukkari dates (weight after seeds removed)
75 ml filtered water
15 ml lemon juice
15 g coconut sugar powdered
8 g virgin coconut oil melted
7 g miso
15 g tahini
1/8 tsp licorice salt from Saltverk (or use pink himalayan salt)

Instructions
Place the dates and water in the Blendtec Twister Jar or a high speed blender. Blend until paste.
Then add the rest of ingredients. Continue to blend until silky smooth.
Transfer mixture in a glass jar. Store in the refrigerator until use. You can use it as a filling in buns.

FIKA

(fee-ka) Swedish

A moment to slow down,
enjoy quality time alone or with friends,
with a cup of your favorite drink
and pastries.

MOROTSKAKA

SWEDISH CARROT CAKE

Time - 1 hour prep + 2 hours setting
Serves - 6 slices

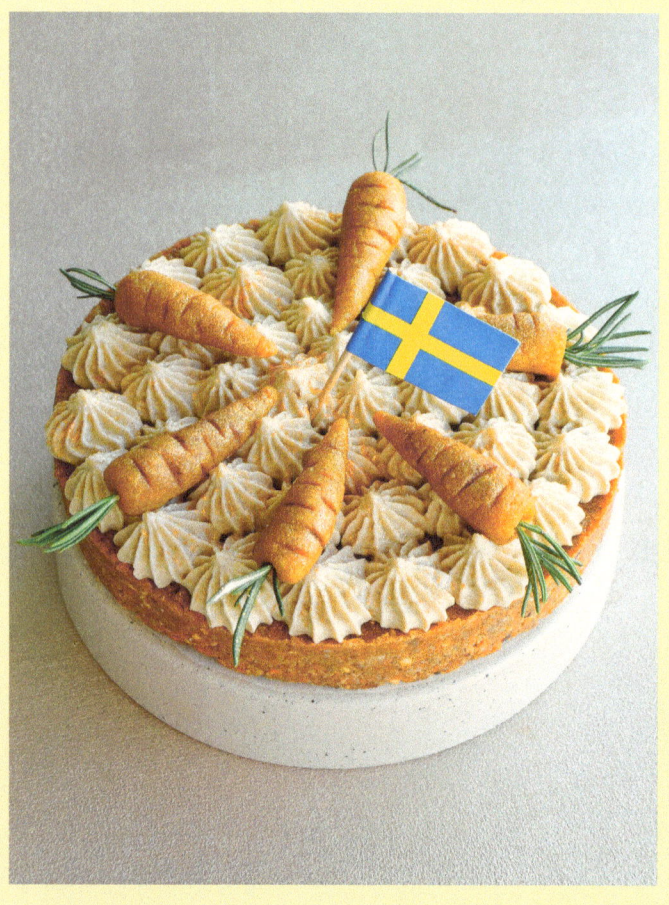
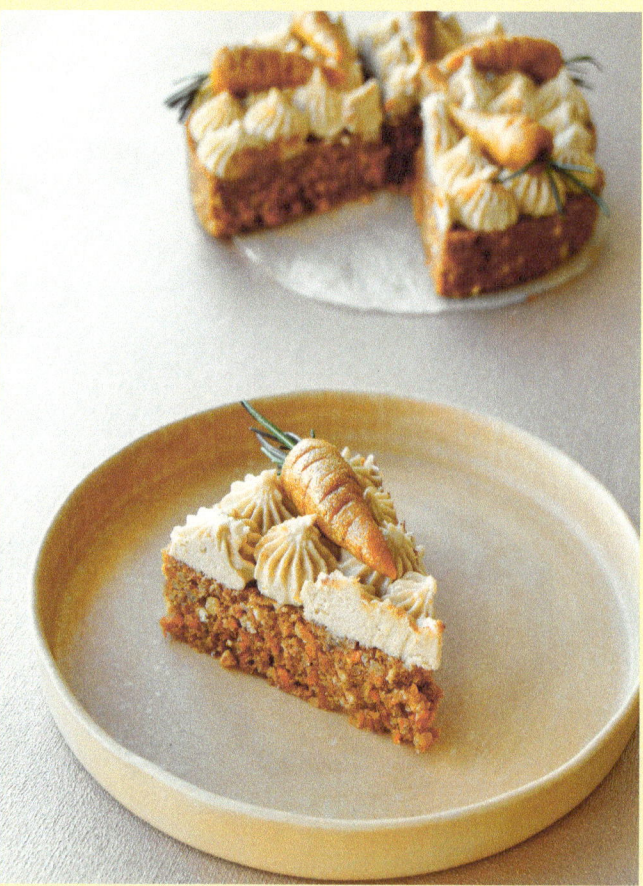

Morotskaka which means carrot cake - A Swedish cake based on carrots and very spicy nuts, as it involves the addition of ginger and cinnamon, traditionally covered, and sometimes even stuffed, with a glaze prepared with fresh spreadable cheese and lemon flavored icing sugar. In our raw version, you will enjoy sunflower cheesecream with flavoured orange and maple.

Crust
150 g shredded carrots
20 g walnuts
65 g brazil nuts
50 g buckini
15 g coconut flour
65 g coconut sugar
6 g shredded fresh ginger
15 ml coconut oil melted
10 ml raw cacao butter melted
15 g psyllium husk powder
2-3 drops of orange essential oil
30 ml lemon juice
3 g cinnamon powder
3 g cardamom powder
5 g vanilla powder

Sunflower Cheese Frosting
120 g sunflower seeds soaked
12 g nutritional yeast (optional)
22 g melted raw cacao butter
60 g maple syrup
60 ml water
60 ml lemon juice
5 ml vanilla extract

Marzipan Carrots
100 g almond flour
50 ml maple syrup
8 g turmeric + 4 g paprika
(you can also use gojiberries or carrot to color the marzipan)
Fresh rosemary to decorate

CRUST
Place shredded carrots, fresh ginger and lemon juice in the food processor, mix together until puree. Then add rest of the ingredients except psyllium. Process again. Lastly add the psyllium husk powder and mix well until everything combined well. Let the dough sit for 5-10 minutes until psyllium absorbs all the water content and you get a sticky thick dough that holds together. Place the mixture in a 15x15 cm cake mould. Press well to flatten out. Let it sit in the refrigerator while making the frosting.

SUNFLOWER CHEESE FROSTING
Place the soaked and strained sunflower seeds in a blender. Add the rest of ingredients except cacao butter. Blend together and smooth. Lastly add melted cacao butter. Blend well.

MARZIPAN CARROTS
To make marzipan carrots, place the almond flour and maple in a bowl. Knead with your hands until dough comes together. Then add the powders and knead again. Let it sit in the refrigerator for 1 hour or in the freezer for 30 minutes before shaping.
Divide the dough between small balls. Give them a carrot shape with your hands. Using the end of a knife dipped in raw cacao powder, make 5-6 short and long, different slits on the carrots marzipans. Decorate the dips with rosemary. Freeze for 30 minutes.

ASSEMBLY
Remove the crust from the refrigerator. Pour the frosting over the cake. Spread well. You can alternatively pipe the cream over the cake in dots or desired shape. Refrigerate again until the frosting is thick enough, for about 2-3 hours. Once marzipan carrots are chilled for 30 minutes then carefully place them over the cake. Slice and serve the cake.

KITKAT PRALINE BARS

Time - 30 minutes prep + 40 minutes setting
Serves - 8-10 slices

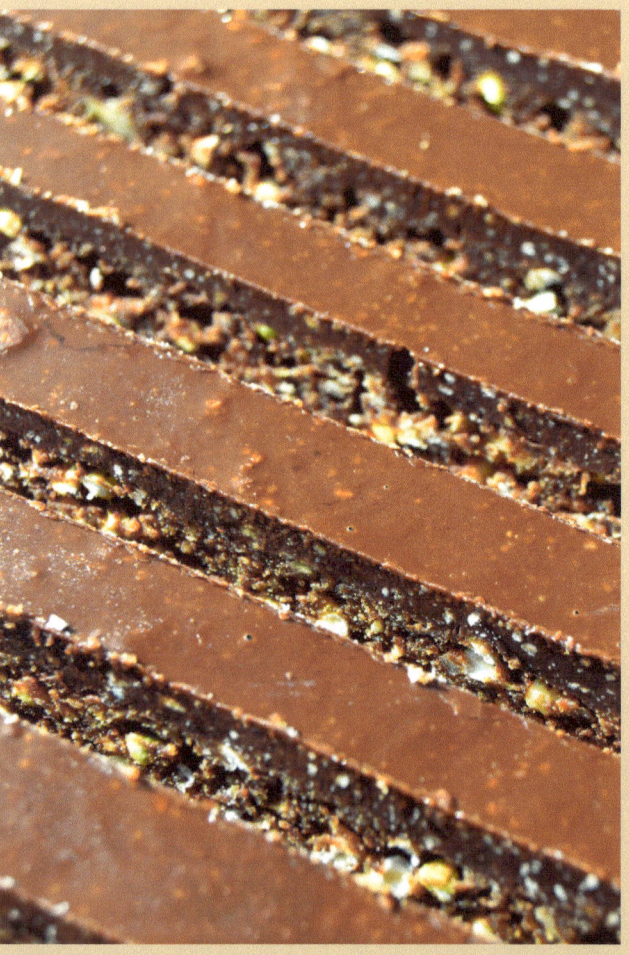
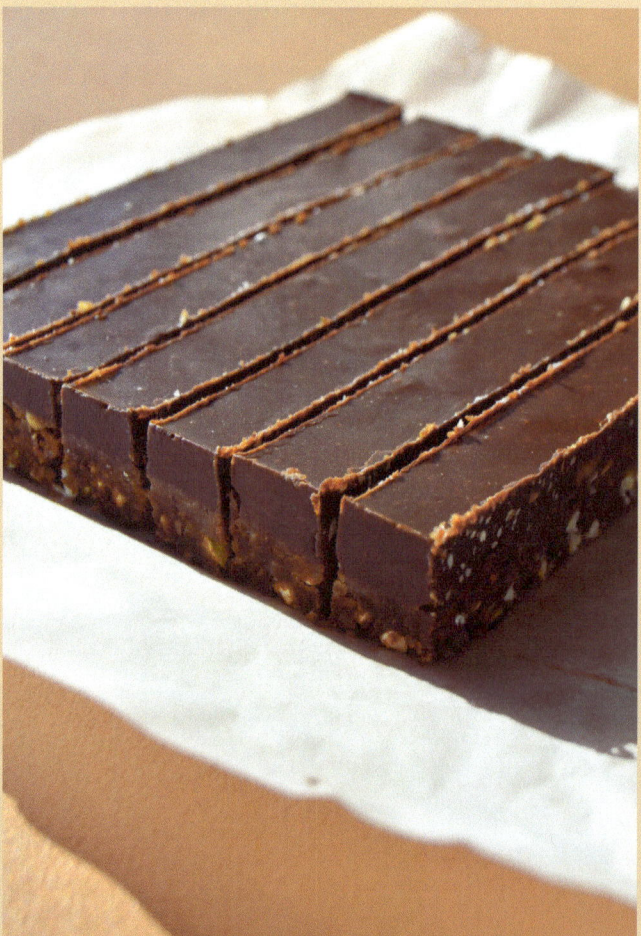

Nothing tickles the memory buds like a childhood experience.
And who can forget childhood treats like Toblerone, KitKat and Ferrero Rocher, among others that were the answer to all our sugar cravings as a young humanbeing unconsciously. As an adult, you can now relive those childhood memories with our tantalisingly raw sweets sprinkled with some fairy dust and a healthy dose of nostalgia. These indulgent raw chocolate hazelnut wafer cakes are perfect answer for KitKats.

Wafer Crust
60 g hazelnut flour
50 g buckini (activated dehydrated buckwheat groats - page 17)
20 ml virgin coconut oil melted
15 g coconut flour
40 g coconut sugar powdered
15 ml maple syrup
35 ml coconut milk
10 g raw cacao powder
7.5 ml tamari or coconut aminos (for soy-free)

Praline
60 g hazelnut butter
60 g raw chocolate (page 28)
15 ml virgin coconut oil melted
A pinch of pink himalayan salt

WAFER CRUST
Place the hazelnut flour, buckini, coconut flour, coconut sugar and raw cacao in a mixing bowl, mix together.
Then add the water, melted coconut oil and coconut aminos.
Using a spoon mix everything well.
Knead the dough with your hands.
Line a 15×15 cm square baking tin lined parchment paper.
Press down the dough in the tin, flatten out.

PRALINE
Using baine marie method, melt the raw chocolate at 42°C, then add the hazelnut butter, salt and coconut oil, mix together until smooth.
Pour mixture over the wafer crust layer.
Freeze for 30-40 minutes. Then remove from the tin.
Using a sharp chef knife, cut the cake carefully into 10 equal long slices. Serve as naked or sprinkle some raw cacao nibs on top if desired.

RAW FIKA RECIPES

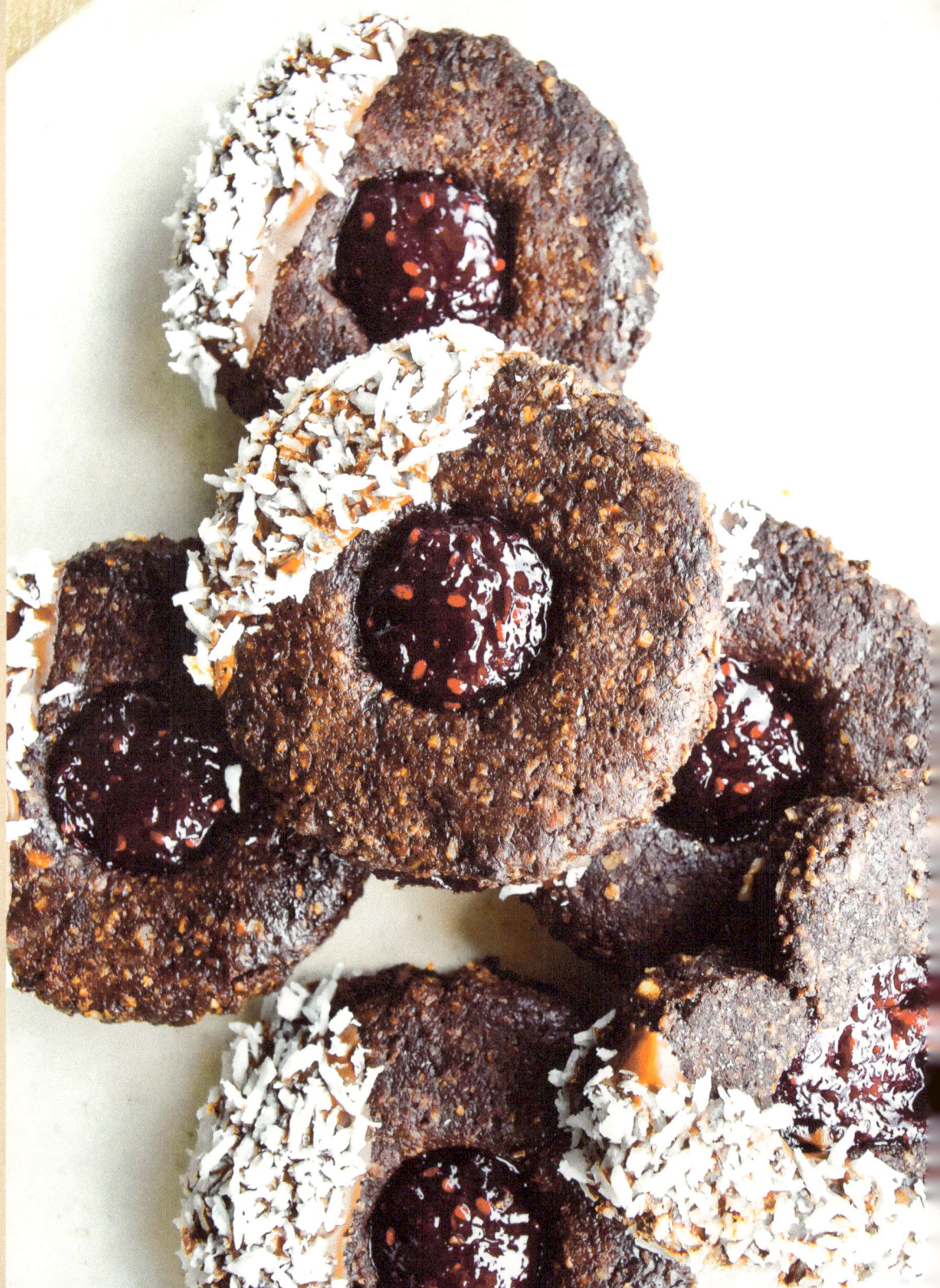

RAW FIKA

SINGOALLA

CHEWY CHOCOLATE COOKIES WITH RASPBERRY

Singoalla - A Swedish equivalent to Tim Tams, with a shortbread biscuit with raspberry, citrus, licorice or blueberry filling and cream with vanilla flavour. In our version we used one of favorite raw cookie base we have developed, matched with vibrant raspberry jam, dipped in raw chocolate and topped with desiccated coconut.

Time - 2 hours + 6-8 hrs dehydration
Serves - 6-8 cookies

Cookies

8 g chia seeds + 60 ml water
88 g sprouted oat flour
56 g hazelnut flour
25 g raw cacao powder
15 g coconut sugar
60 ml maple syrup
65 g hazelnut butter
15 ml extra virgin olive oil
2 g licorice salt from Saltverk or pink himalayan salt
2 g baking soda
40 g chopped raw chocolate

Cherry Jam

200 g defrosted cherries
60 ml maple syrup
7 g chia seeds

Decoration

25 g desiccated coconut
60 g melted raw chocolate (page 28 or use packaged one of your choice)

COOKIES

To make cookies, in a mixing bowl, mix chia seeds and water. Keep stirring for the first minute or so to prevent the chia seeds from clumping together. Then set aside for 5 minutes.

Add the rest of ingredients in the chia seed mixture. Stir well to combine. Fold in the finely chopped chocolate.

Place the bowl in the freezer for 15 minutes. You will be able to work easier with the dough now. Roll it out between two pieces of parchment paper about 1/4 inch thickness. Cut them with a 2-3 inch cookie cutter. Dampen the cutter between cuts to keep it cutting clean and not sticking to the dough. Continue the process till all dough is used. Then cut a small hole in the middle with a smaller cutter. Transfer the cookies onto a baking tray lined parchment paper. Dehydrate for 8 hours or until both sides of the cookies are fully dried.

CHERRY JAM

Place defrosted cherries and maple in a blender. process until puree. Pass through a sieve, remove the pulp. Transfer the rest to a bowl, add the chia seeds. Dehydrate at 42°C for 5-6 or until thick enough.

ASSEMBLY

Once cookies are done, spoon 1-2 tsp jam into the middle of the cookie and lightly spread it out to cover 3/4 of the cookie. Leaving just a little room on the edge of the cookie all around. Place a cookie with a hole in it on top and gently press so the jam comes out the top a little and just reaches the sides of the cookie. Place the tray of cookies into the dehydrator to dry with the jam for 1 hour or until they have reached the firmness you desire. Once done, you could let them cool and then dip the tops or sides in chocolate and then dip in the desiccated coconut or just keep them as is. These will store well at room temp for 2 days or in an airtight container in the fridge for a week or so.

RAW FIKA

CHOKLADBOLLSEMLA

CHOCOLATE BALL SEMLA

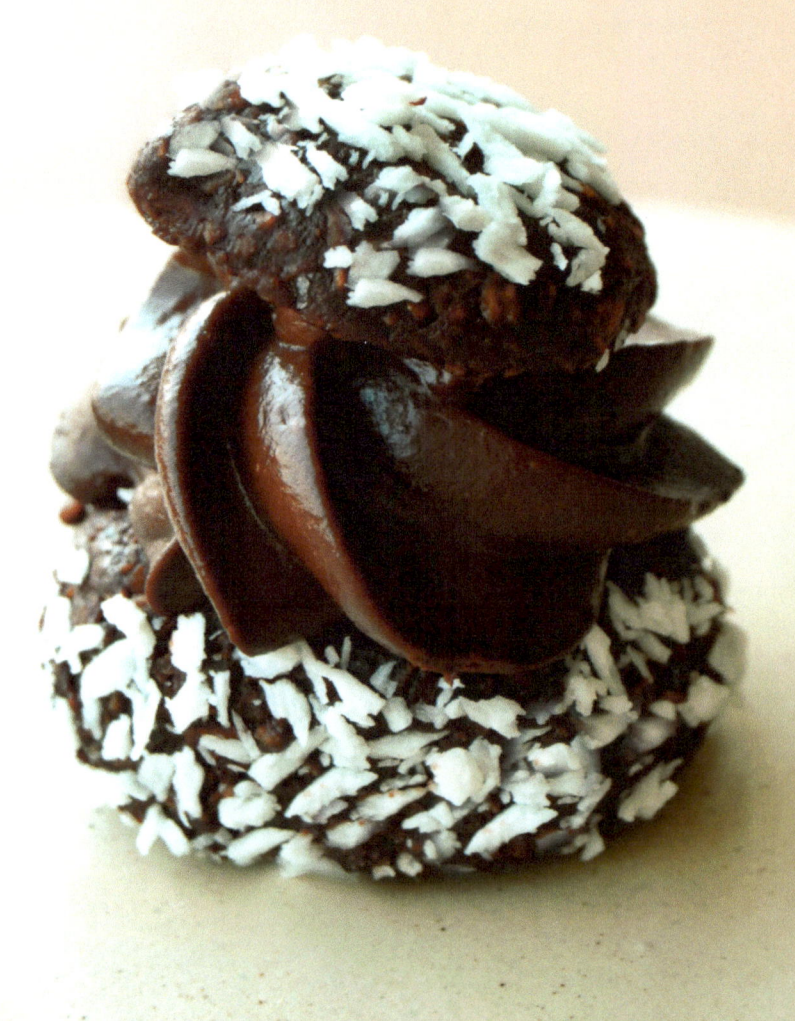

Where the raw semla meets raw chokladboll. The idea of mixing the two most lovable Swedish pastries of all time? This intense version of chokladboll filled with delicious avocado chocolate cream would be your new favourite.
In Sweden, there is a day just celebrating the chokladbollar on May 11th every year.

Time - 40 min prep + 2 hours setting
Serves - makes 10 balls

Chokladboll Dough
100 g gluten-free rolled oats or sprouted oat flour (page 16-17)
50 g desiccated coconut
15 ml cold press coconut oil melted
50 g raw chocolate melted
35 g coconut sugar powdered
7 g raw cacao powder
45 ml cold press coffee
A pinch of pink himalayan salt

Avocado Chocolate Cream
100 g ripe avocado (weight after seed and skin removed)
50 g raw chocolate melted
15 ml maple syrup

Topping
30 g desiccated coconut

CHOKLADBOLL DOUGH
Melt the raw chocolate and coconut oil together using bain marie method.
Meanwhile, put the oats and coconut sugar in a high speed blender. Process until combined and almost in powder form.
Then add the raw cacao powder and salt, blend to combine together.
Pour the melted raw chocolate, coconut oil and coffee over the mixture. Mix everything until the dough perfectly holds together. You'll see big ball in the food processor when it starts to get a dough shape.
Then remove from the food processor. Make 10 balls with your hands.

AVOCADO CHOCOLATE CREAM
To make avocado chocolate cream, place the avocado in the food processor, add the melted raw chocolate and maple syrup, blender together. Let it cool in the fridge for 1-2 hours. Then transfer to a piping bag with your favorite nozzle.

ASSEMBLY
Assemble your semla balls by cutting of the top of balls, don't cut it in half. It should be a bun and small top.
Set the tops aside, fill the bun with avocado chocolate cream by piping the cream on top.
Put the top on the cream and sprinkle some desiccated or coconut flour on top.

RAW FIKA

KANELBULLE

CINNAMON BUN WITH DATE CARAMEL

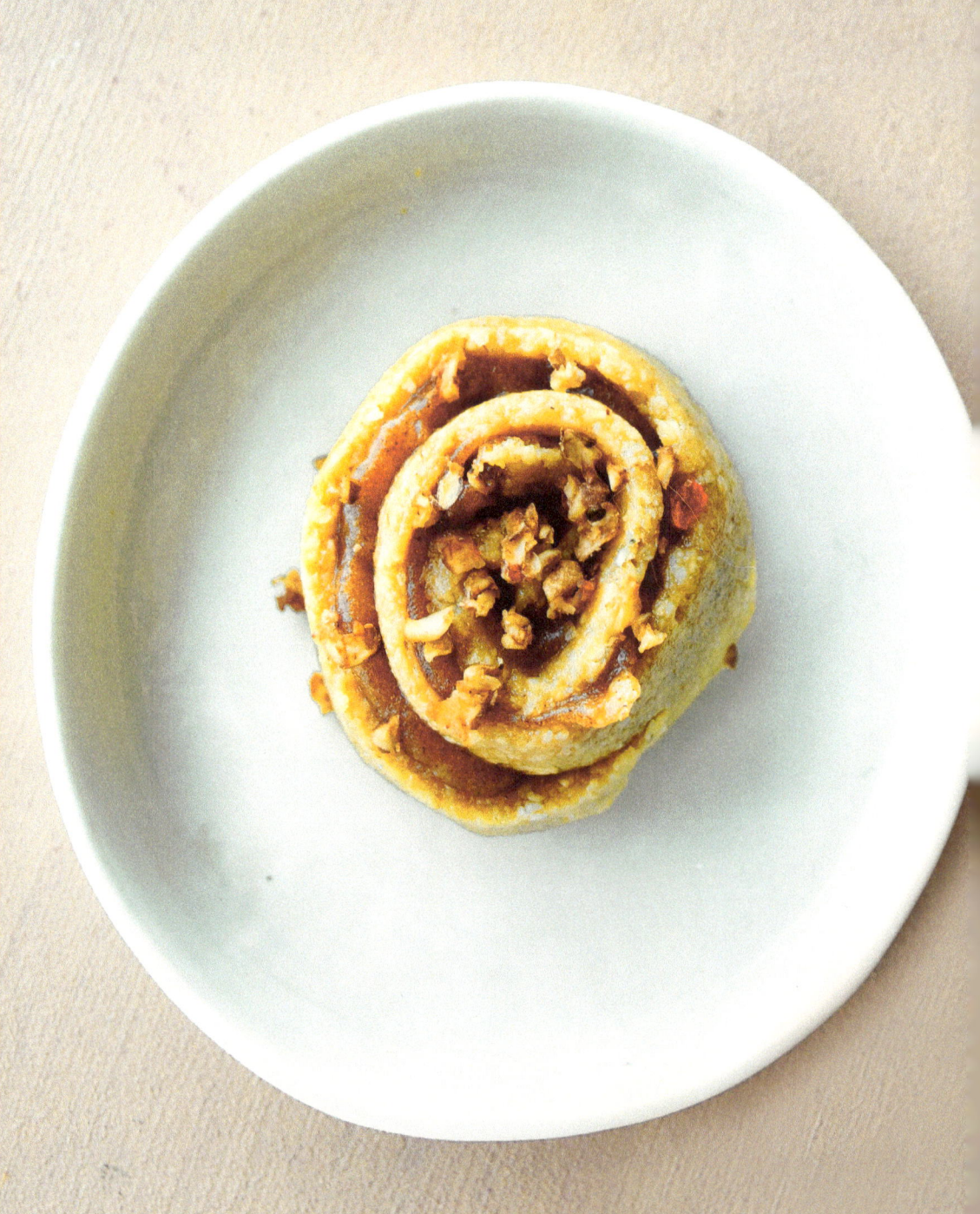

In Sweden we take fika and baked goods very seriously (particularly cinnamon buns.) I wanted a healthier alternative to the traditional cinnamon bun, and that's how I ended up with this sweet. Delicious and guilt-free, what a dream come true.

Time - 1 hour prep + 4 hours dehydration
Serves - makes 2 trays

Bun Dough
90 g oat flour
100 g almond flour
50 ml maple syrup
20 ml virgin coconut oil melted
5 g ground cardamom
A pinch pink himalayan salt
15 ml water as needed

Cinnamon Filling
1 batch homemade raw date caramel (page 31)
50 g dried raisins
15 ml virgin coconut oil melted
7 g cinnamon powder
A pinch of pink himalayan salt

Celeriac Almond Crumb
200 g celeriac
50 g finely chopped almonds
15 g coconut sugar
15 ml coconut aminos
1/4 tsp red pepper flakes
A pinch pink himalayan salt

CELERIAC ALMOND CRUMB
Make the celeriac almond crumb beforehand.
Peel and wash your celeriac. Transfer in a food processor, blend until you get rice-like texture.
Squeeze them with your hands and remove the excess water. Transfer to a bowl. Add the coconut aminos, salt, coconut sugar, almonds and pepper. Mix to combine together.
Spread on a dehydrator sheet lined parchment paper. Dehydrate at 42°C for 3-4 hours or until fully dried.

CINNAMON FILLING
Place the date caramel in a bowl. Add the rest of the ingredients listed under cinnamon filling in the caramel.
Mix well until well combined. Taste and adjust the salt and cinnamon if needed.

BUN DOUGH
Place the almond flour and all remaining ingredients in a food processor and mix into a dough. Freeze for 15 minutes.

ASSEMBLY
Roll out between two baking sheets to a rectangle shape. Spread the cinnamon filling on the dough and cut strips about 2 cm wide with a sharp chef knife. Roll up each strip and give them a smaller bun shape. Sprinkle the celeriac almond crumb on top of the buns. Set them in the fridge for an hour or so before serving.

SEMLA
WITH RASPBERRY JAM, CARAMEL AND CREAM

Time - 3 hours prep + 6 hrs dehydration + 1 hour setting
Serves - 9 buns

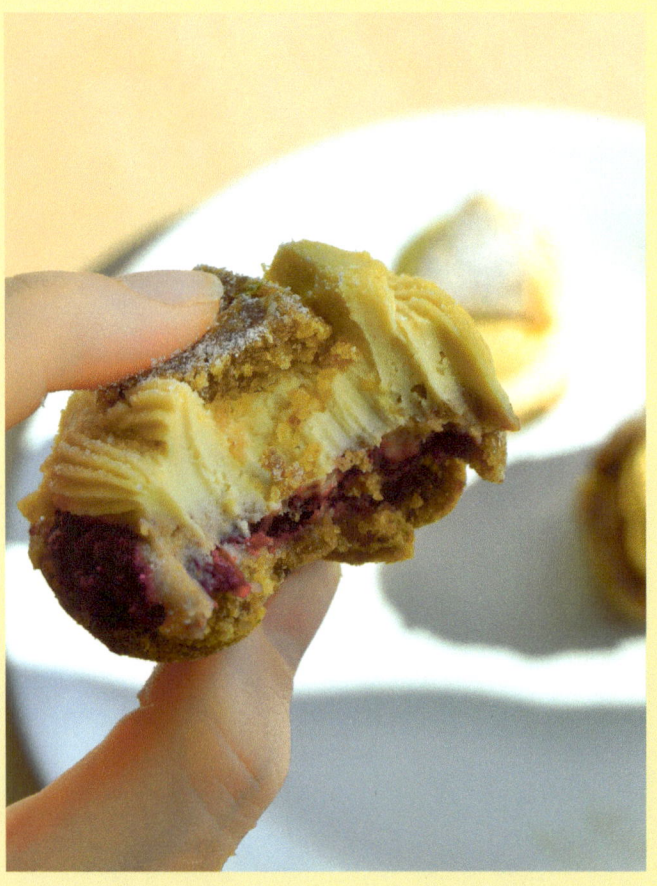
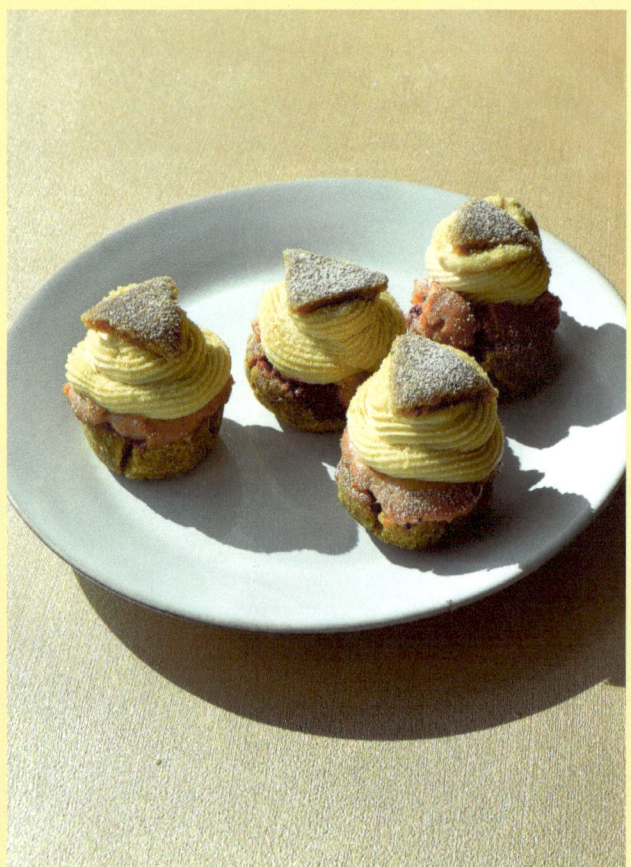

Semla aka fastlagsbulle has one of the richer histories of Swedish. A semla bun is a soft roll that's been hollowed and had its top removed, filled with almond paste and whipped cream, then re-topped and dusted with sugar. Originally, they were only eaten on "Fat Tuesday" (Fettisdag : the day before the Lent fast) but now they can be found in bakeries from end of January through Easter. Eat these the traditional Swedish way and use the top to scoop out the filling.

Bun Dough
Dry Ingredients
140 g almond flour
20 g coconut flour
20 g psyllium husk powder
22 g ground flaxseed
4 g cardamom powder
1/2 tsp pink himalayan salt

Wet Ingredients
200 g zucchini
90 g medjool dates soaked
40 ml lemon juice

Almond Date Caramel
75 g medjool dates (weight after pitted)
70 g almond butter
50 g coconut cream
30 ml virgin coconut oil melted
15 ml maple syrup
7 ml tamari or coconut aminos

White Cream
1 batch coconut frosting or white chocolate frosting of your choice (page 26)

Raspberry Jam
1 batch raspberry jam (page 29)

Decoration
Coconut flour or erythritol for dusting

Before you start, make sure you prepared raspberry jam and white chocolate frosting beforehand.

BUN DOUGH
Peel your zucchini, cut into small chunks and add to your food processor. Squeeze the lemon over the zucchini. Then add soaked and rinsed medjool dates. Process until puree. Add all dry ingredients. Continue to mix the zucchini date puree and dry ingredients together until you have a fine dough that sticks together. If the dough feels wet, add 1 tsp buckini flour at a time or if feels dry, add more lemon juice. Knead the dough with your hands and divide between 9 equal pieces. Then roll the pieces into small balls. Put them on your dehydrator tray, press so that they stand firmly and dehydrate in the dehydrator at 42°C for about 6 hours or until you feel that they are a little firm on the outside. They should not be too dry but have a core that is juicy. Carefully cut the top off the buns, then shape in the triangle using a sharp knife. Using a small teaspoon or apple core remover, dig the core out a little. Place the lids and buns on the dehydrator sheet, continue to dehydrate for additional 2 hours.

ALMOND FILLING
To make almond filling cream, pour the almond butter in the blender, add the rest of ingredients, whisk well until slightly becomes thicken. Set in the refrigerator during the dehydration process of buns.

ASSEMBLY
Once buns are done, remove them from the dehydrator. Remove the almond cream from the refrigerator. Place 2 tsp raw raspberry jam in the hollows. Freeze for 30 minutes. Then put 2 tsp almond cream filling on the raspberry jam layer. Freeze again for 30 minutes. Using a piping bag with desired nozzle, pipe the white cream over the jam. Put the lid of bun. Sprinkle some coconut flour or erythritol if desired. Enjoy!

RAW FIKA

SMULPAJ

APPLE CRUMBLE PIE

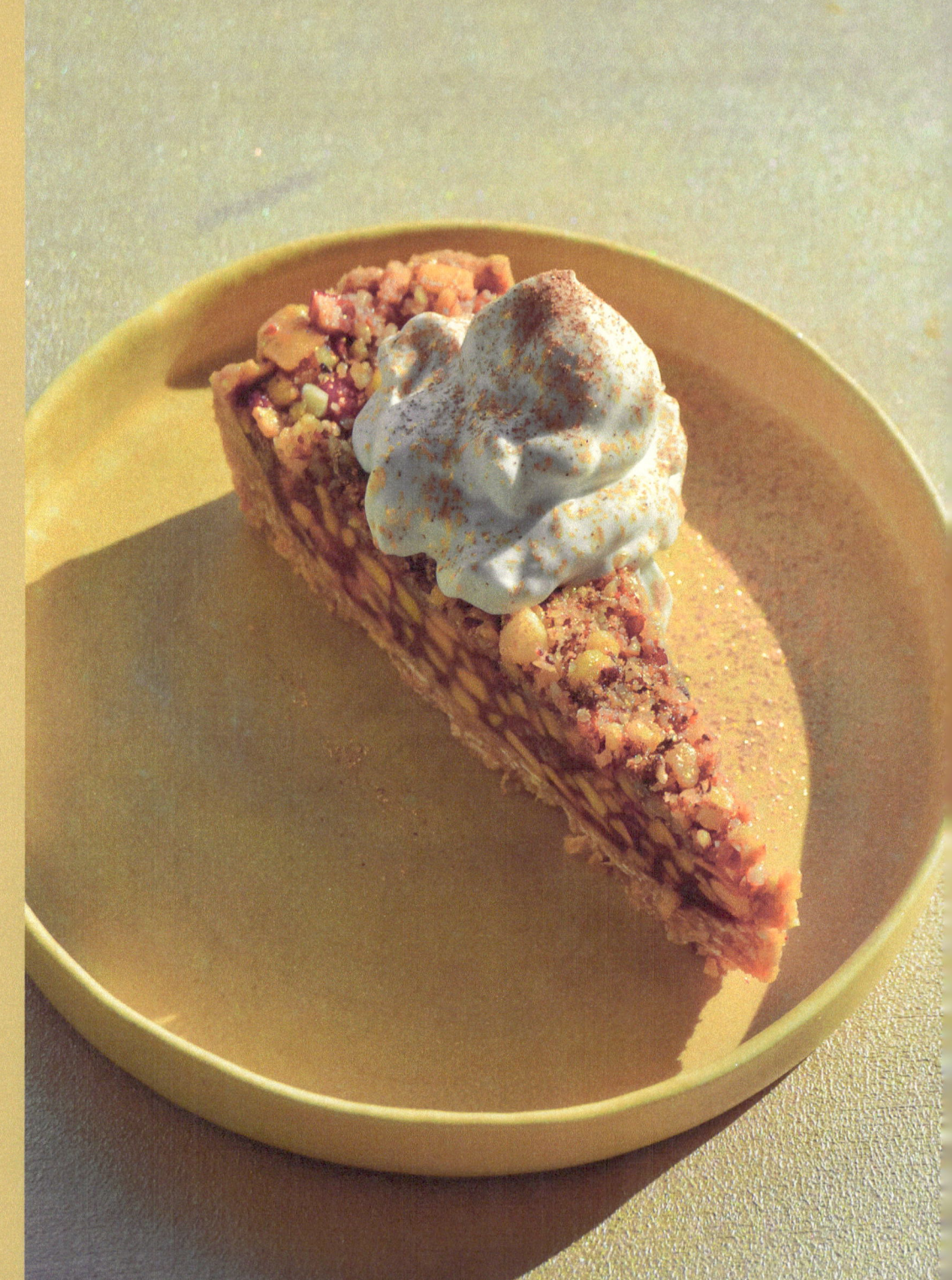

A sign of autumn: Swedish Smulpaj.

It's a delicious combination of cake, cookie and pie with seasonal fruits and so simple to make! Smulpaj differs from traditional pies in that it has no pastry shell; instead, fillings are added directly to the pie.

In Sweden, it is made with almonds or oats. So naturally gluten-free. The filling is commonly made with apples, rhubarb, or bilberries, and served with whipped cream, vanilla sauce, or ice cream.

Time - 30 min prep + 1 hour setting
Serves - 10 cm x 2 pies

Tart dough

130 g oat flour
55 g almond flour
25 g desiccated coconut
25 g almond butter
20 ml virgin coconut oil melted
60 ml maple syrup
20 ml oat milk
1/8 tsp pink himalayan salt

Apple Filling

200 g ripe red apple, cored
80 g coconut sugar
35 g dried raisins, soaked
15 g grated ginger
7 g psyllium husk powder
1/2 tsp cinnamon powder
1/4 tsp ground cardamom
1/8 tsp ground clove
1/8 tsp ground nutmeg
A pinch pink himalayan salt

Top Crumble

50 g chopped walnuts
30 g coconut sugar
2 drops bergamot essential oil
1 drop rosemary essential oil
A pinch of pink himalayan salt

TART DOUGH

Place almond flour, oat flour, desiccated coconut and salt in a food processor, Mix together. Then add maple syrup, coconut oil, almond butter and oat milk. Mix together until comes together. Using your hands knead the dough in the bowl. When it holds together, remove from the bowl.

TOP CRUMBLE

To make top crumble, place all ingredients in a food processor, mix together. Set aside.

ALMOND FILLING

To make almond filling, finely dice the apples, place in a large bowl. Add the rest of ingredients, toss together. Let it sit to marinate for 1-2 hours. You can use the filling after marination or you can dehydrate for a soft cooked-like consistency. To dehydrate, place them in the dehydrator in a bowl for 6 hours at 46°C. Alternatively you can cook the apples sous vide at 46°C. (Sous-vide raw cooking method can be found in our "Mad About Raw" cookbook)

ASSEMBLY

Divide the tart dough between 10 cm small tart tins. Press down and shape with your hands or with a back of spoon. Repeat with the remaining dough. You can also randomly put the dough in the tin instead shaping.

Once apples are cooked, divide the apple filling between tart tins. Drizzle some of the leftover juice if have any. Add the top crumble to coat the apple layer.

Serve with whippped coconut cream if desired.

RAW FIKA

DAMMSUGARE

SWEDISH VACUUM CLEANER

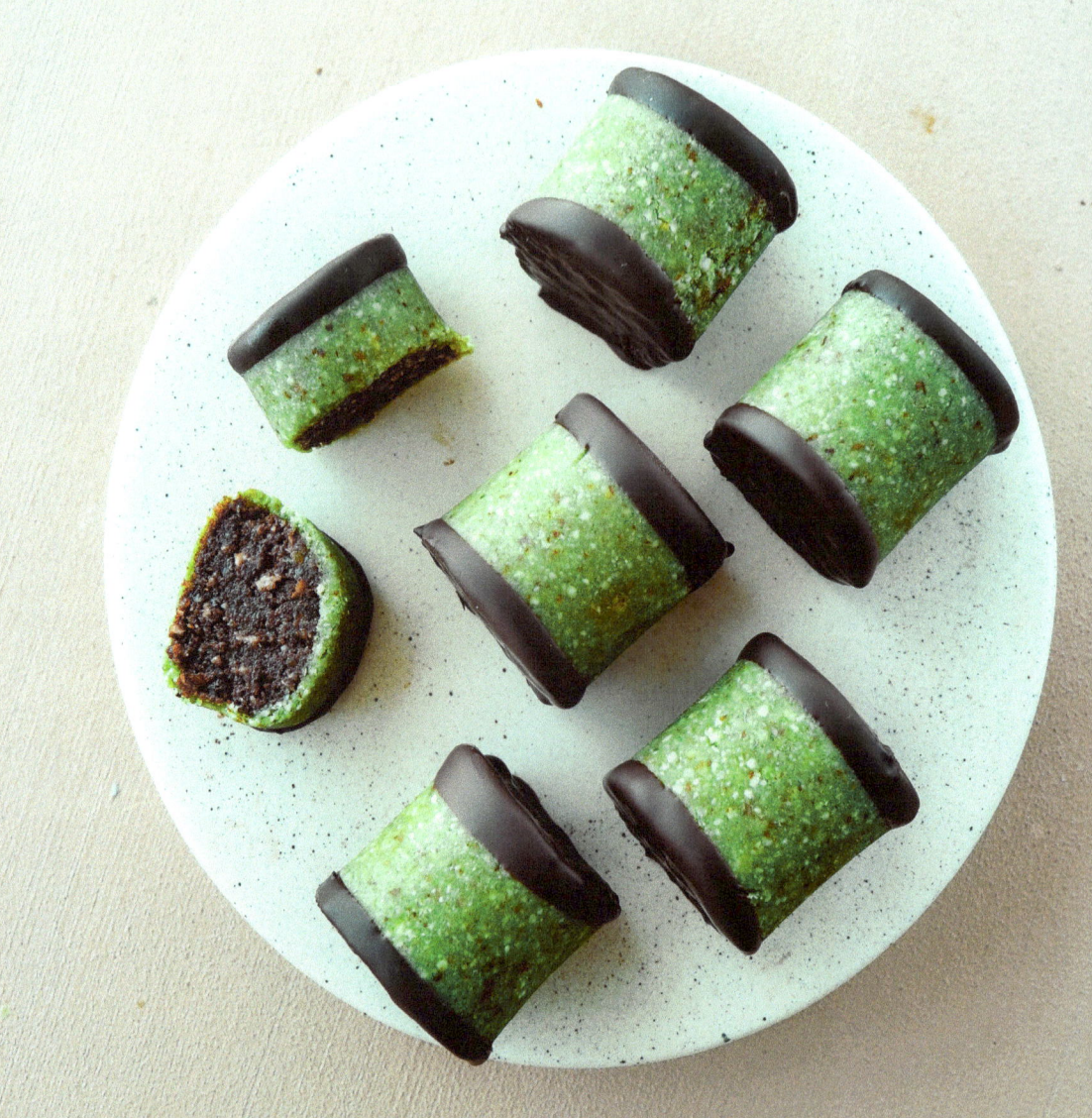

Swedish Dammsugare is one of Sweden's most loved pastries. It is a small, cylinder rolled in green marzipan with both ends dipped in chocolate and it is filled with a soft, sweet arrack flavored punsch dough. They first became a thing when bakers needed to find a way of using yesterdays cake crumbs, mixed with a bit of sugar and liqueur for flavour. Today they are amongst the most popular sweet treats in Sweden. Our raw version is a healthy twist on a classic.

Time - 2 hours prep + 2 hours setting
Serves - 12 - 16 pieces

Green Marzipan
15 g fresh collard greens or spinach
100 g almond flour
100 ml maple syrup or coconut nectar
35 g coconut flour
1/4 tsp spirulina powder
1/8 tsp turmeric powder

Chocolate Punsch Dough
100 g activated dehydrated almond flour
130 g soft medjool dates (weight after pitted)
35 g desiccated coconut
30 g raw cacao powder
20 ml virgin coconut oil melted
5 ml arrack extract or essence
1/4 tsp licorice salt

Chocolate Dipping
100 g raw cacao mass
15 ml maple syrup
8 ml virgin coconut oil melted
5 ml vanilla extract

OR

melt and use your favorite raw chocolate for dipping - 100 g

GREEN MARZIPAN
Start by blending the maple and spinach in a high speed blender until you have a smooth green sauce. Then strain the mixture and remove the pulp (the biggest pieces from the spinach).
Transfer the spinach maple sauce to a bowl. Add the turmeric and spirulina, whisk well. Then add the almond flour slowly while blending. When the paste is too thick to blend, move it to a bowl and work the dough with your hands while adding the coconut flour until you get a very firm dough with marzipan texture.
When the marzipan is done move it to a baking paper and fold another baking paper on top, roll the dough flat with a rolling pin and let it rest on the baking paper while you make the punsch dough.

CHOCOLATE PUNSCH DOUGH
Blend all ingredients for the punsch dough in a food processor and blend until you have a dough with the same texture as raw balls. Make three long rolls of the punsch dough and place one on top of the green marzipan and fold it in. Then cut and roll to smooth. Repeat the process for the rest. Keep in the freezer for 15-20 minutes before cutting to get smooth nice shape.

ASSEMBLY
Using a ruller, cut 3 inch long punch rolls and set them aside while melting the chocolate.
Melt the cacao solid in a dehydrator, add the rest of the ingredients when the chocolate is melted and whisk it slowly with a spoon. Dip one side of the punsch roll at the time, on the parchment paper set aside in the fridge for about 10-15 minutes to solidify. Then dip another side of the punsch roll. Refrigerate again at least 15-20 minutes before serving.

CITRON PUNSCHROLL

I always hear that how difficult to find arrack for those who live outside Sweden. In this recipe, we created a new healthy raw dammsugare with lemon flavour and turmeric without using arrack. So you can easily make it without Swedish ingredients now! Hope you enjoy as much as we do.

Time - 2 hours prep + 2 hours setting
Serves - 12 - 16 pieces

Citron Marzipan
3 g turmeric
100 g activated dehydrated almond flour
25 g sprouted buckwheat flour
60 ml maple syrup or coconut nectar
10 ml lemon extract or 4-5 drops of lemon essential oil

Chocolate Dipping
100 g raw cacao mass
15 ml maple syrup
8 ml virgin coconut oil melted
5 ml vanilla extract

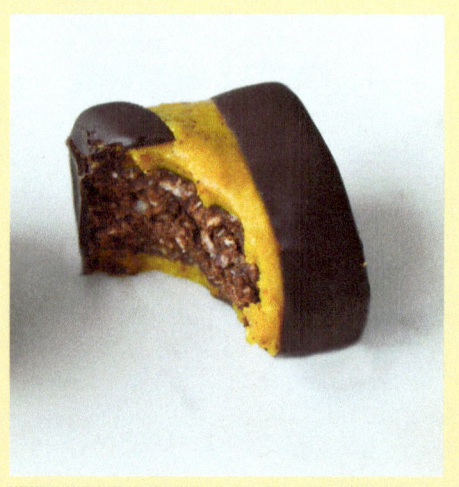

Chocolate Punsch Dough
50 g activated dehydrated almond flour
50 g sprouted rolled oat flour
35 g desiccated coconut
30 g raw cacao powder
70 g maple syrup
20 g virgin coconut oil melted
1/4 tsp pink himalayan salt

CITRON MARZIPAN
Place almond flour, buckwheat flour and turmeric in a bowl, mix together. Then add maple syrup and lemon extract, mix well using a spoon. When the marzipan is done transfer it to a baking paper and place another baking paper on top, roll the dough flat using a rolling pin and let it cool in the fridge while making punsch dough.

CHOCOLATE PUNSCH DOUGH
Blend all ingredients for the punsch dough in a food processor and blend until you have a dough with the same texture as raw balls. Make three long rolls of the punsch dough and place one on top of the citron marzipan and fold it in. Then cut and roll to smooth. Repeat the process for the rest. Keep in the freezer for 15-20 minutes before cutting to get smooth nice shape.

ASSEMBLY
To assemble the punschrolls, follow the same instructions given on the previous page for the green dammsugare.

BOUNTY PUNSCHROLL

Time - 2 hours prep + 2 hours setting
Serves - 12 - 16 pieces

Coconut Punsch Dough
50 g activated dehydrated cashew flour
50 g sprouted rolled oat flour
35 g desiccated coconut
30 g coconut milk powder
70 ml maple syrup
20 ml virgin coconut oil melted
10 g raw cacao butter melted
1/4 tsp pink himalayan salt
3-4 drops coconut essential oil or extract

Chocolate Dipping
100 g raw chocolate melted (page 28)
8 ml virgin coconut oil melted
Desiccated coconut for the ends

Chocolate Marzipan
100 g activated dehydrated almond flour
25 g coconut flour
35 g raw chocolate melted
60 ml maple syrup or coconut nectar
7 g raw cacao powder
3 g charcoal powder

CHOCOLATE MARZIPAN

Place almond flour, coconut flour, cacao powder and charcoal in a bowl, mix together. Then add maple syrup and melted raw chocolate, mix well using a spoon. When the marzipan is done transfer it to a baking paper and place another baking paper on top, roll the dough flat using a rolling pin and let it cool in the fridge while making punsch dough.

COCONUT PUNSCH DOUGH

Blend all ingredients for the punsch dough in a food processor and blend until you have a dough with the same texture as raw balls. Make three long rolls of the punsch dough and place one on top of the chocolate marzipan and fold it in. Then cut and roll to smooth. Repeat the process for the rest. Keep in the freezer for 15-20 minutes before cutting to get smooth nice shape.

ASSEMBLY

To assemble the punschrolls, follow the same instructions given on the previous page for the green dammsugare. Once dipped the ends in the melted raw chocolate mixed with coconut oil, then dip in desiccated coconut. Allow to cool in the fridge for 20 minutes before serving.

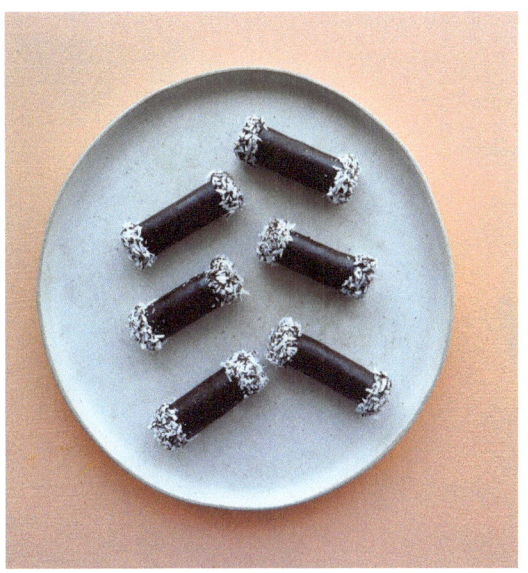

RAW FIKA

CHOKLADSNITTAR

SWEDISH CHOCOLATE COOKIES

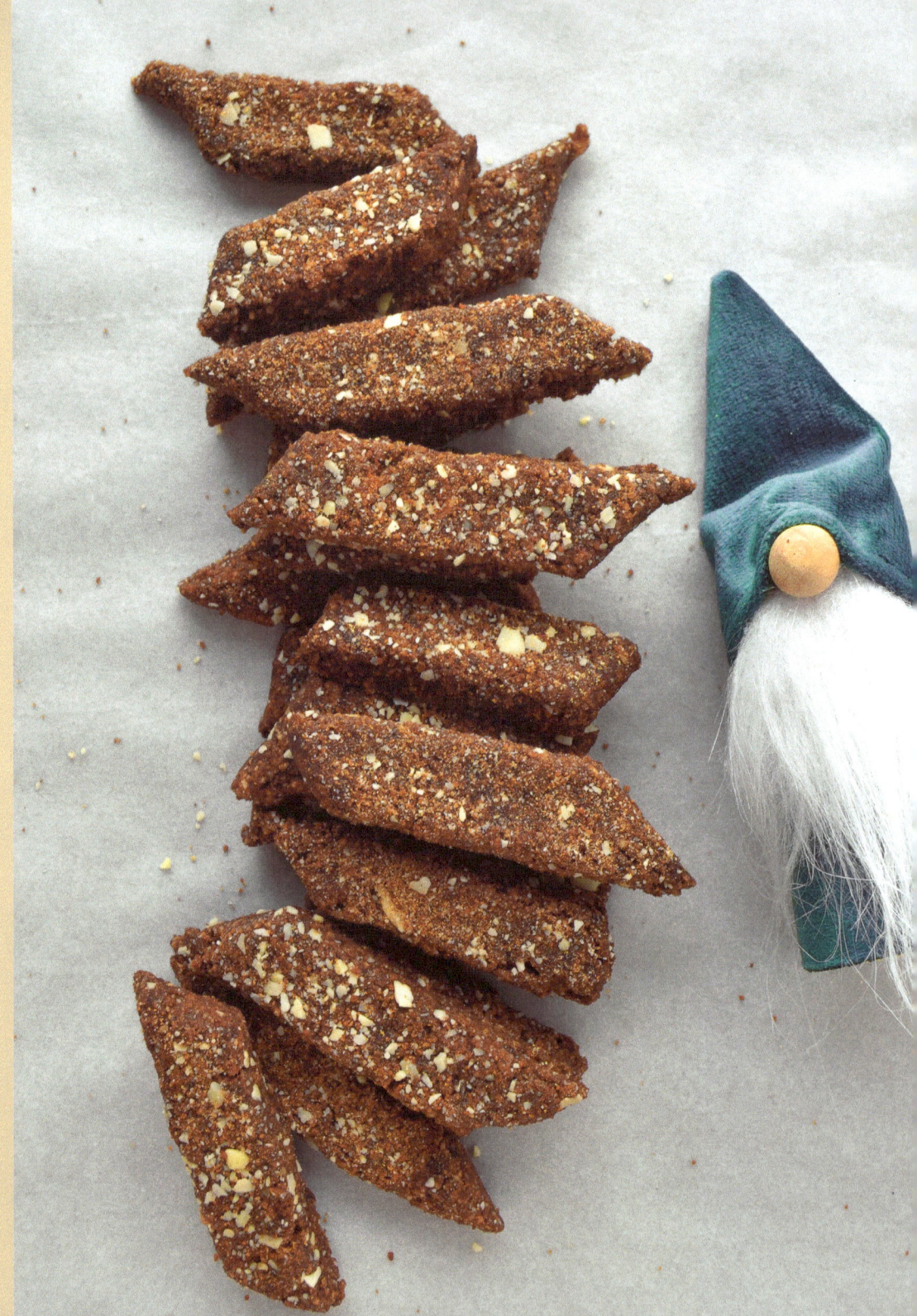

In Sweden there is a thing called "sju sorters småkakor" or seven little cookies.

As much as the etiquette required you to have a lower limit of seven cookies on the cookie plate when your guests come over, you don't necessarily need to prepare seven types of cookies when people pop over (but grandmothers probably did.) These Swedish Chocolate Cuts, known as "Chokladsnittar" in Sweden are a well-loved classic, just one of sju sorters småkakor. Simple to make and full of rich chocolate flavor they are equally suited for everyday fika or holidays. It has a rich taste of chocolate and is chewy. The biggest difference from the the American cookies is maybe the shape. We cut them in diagonal cuts.

Time - 70 minutes prep + 7 hours dehydration
Serves - 6 longs, 36 small cuts

Cookie

8 g chia seeds
60 ml filtered water
45 g sprouted oat flour
45 g almond flour
25 g coconut flour
20 g raw cacao powder
10 g raw coconut sugar powdered
70 g coconut nectar syrup
60 g raw almond butter
15 g melted cacao butter
10 ml extra virgin olive oil
4 g baking soda
5 g tsp ground cardamom
4 g licorice salt or pink himalayan

Toppings

40 g chopped sliced almonds
40 g coconut sugar
5 g vanilla bean powder

COOKIE

In a mixing bowl, mix chia seeds and water. Keep stirring for the first minute or so to prevent the chia seeds from clumping together. Then set aside for 5 minutes.

Then add the rest of ingredients in the chia mixture. Stir well to combine. Place the bowl in the freezer for 20 minutes. Once time is up, remove from the freezer. You will be able to work easier with the dough now. Knead the dough and make a big ball. Then divide into 6 pieces, and form them into a log. Place on the baking sheet and gently flatten them to about a 1/4 inch using your hands or with a help of knife.

TOPPING

In a bowl, mix coconut sugar, vanilla and chopped sliced almonds.

ASSEMBLY

Sprinkle the dough with topping. Cut them on a diagonal, roughly 1 inch wide. In traditional method, they are cut after baking process. Since this is raw method, and we want to decrease the dehydration time, we prefer cutting them beforehand.

Then place in the dehydrator sheet, dehydrate at 42°C for 2 hours or until thick enough. Then flip and continue dehydrating for about 4-5 hours. Once done, you could let them cool before storage. These will store well at room temp for 2 days or in an airtight container in the fridge for a week or so.

RAW FIKA

KANELBULLAR

CINNAMON BUNS WITH CHOCOLATE

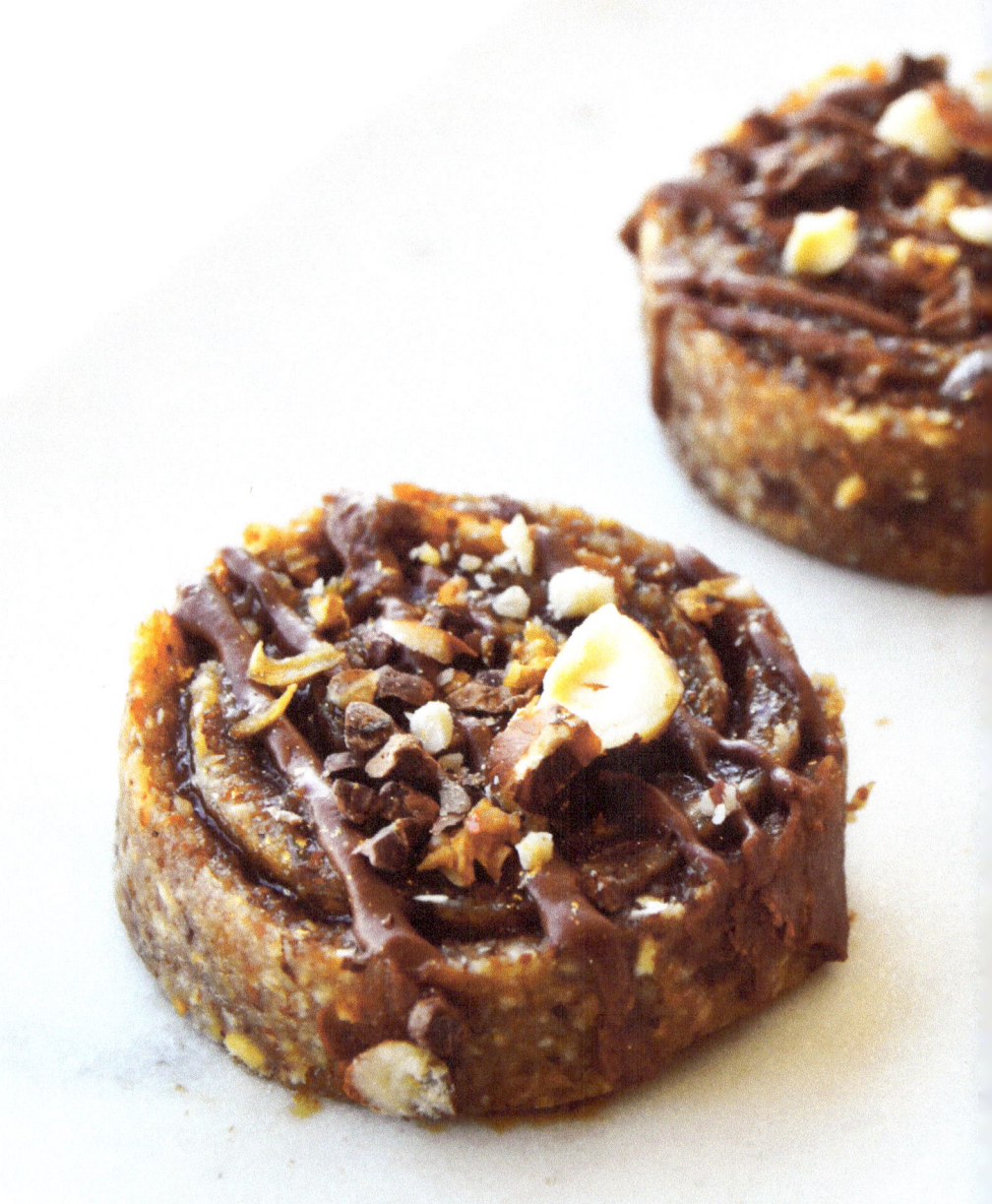

Kanelbullar is definitely one of the most iconic simple Swedish pastries made with basically cinnamon, flour, butter and sugar and is usually present at any fika. Our healthy twist can be made with any nut flour, dried fruits and cinnamon. Cinnamon buns have been around since the 1920s in Sweden and are celebrated on October 4, so mark your calendars for Kanelbullens Dag!

Time - 1 hour prep + 4 hours dehydration
Serves - makes 2 trays

Bun Dough
90 g hazelnut flour
55 g oat flour
100 g raisins
30 ml hazelnut milk
15 ml maple syrup
15 ml virgin coconut oil
4 g ground cardamom
3 g vanilla bean powder
A pinch pink himalayan salt

Cinnamon Filling
1 tsp cinnamon
25 ml virgin coconut oil
15 ml maple syrup
30 g coconut sugar
10 ml tbsp water
A pinch licorice or pink himalayan salt

Chocolate Sauce
30 g coconut oil melted
25 g cup raw cacao powder
25 g coconut sugar powdered (grind in the coffee grinder beforehand)
45 ml filtered water
A pinch of salt

Toppings
Jerusalem artichoke crumb (inst. pg. 43)
Chopped hazelnuts
Raw cacao nibs

BUN DOUGH
Place the flours and the rest of remaining ingredients in a food processor and mix into a dough that holds together.
Roll the dough between two parchment paper in rectangle shape and set in the fridge to cool for about 15 minutes.

CINNAMON FILLING
Place all the ingredients in a small bowl and whisk well until smooth paste.

CHOCOLATE SAUCE
Melt the coconut oil using bain marie method. Transfer to the Blendtec Twister Jar or a high speed blender. Add the rest of ingredients over the coconut oil. Blend well. Ensure coconut sugar is blended enough to remove any grainy texture. Process until emulsified and has thickened.
Pour into a squeeze bottle to use immediately. Otherwise keep in the refrigerator. Let it sit at room temperature before using.

ASSEMBLY
Spread the cinnamon paste thinly on the bun dough.
Refrigerate at least 30 minutes or put in the freezer for 10-15 minutes. Then cut strips about 1 cm wide with a sharp chef knife. Roll up each strip like a bun. Make the Jerusalem artichoke crumb according the instructions given on page 43, just use jerusalem artichokes instead of celeriac. Once dehydrated, mix jerusalem artichoke crumb, chopped hazelnuts and raw cacao nibs together and sprinkle on top of the bun.
Drizzle some chocolate sauce over the buns. (if dehydrating, use after the dehydration process, if refrigerating, use before sitting in the fridge)

Option 1: Set the buns in the dehydrator at 42°C for 4 hours.
Option 2: Skip the baking and set them in the fridge for an hour or so before serving.

RAW FIKA

BROWNIE
WITH COCONUT BACON

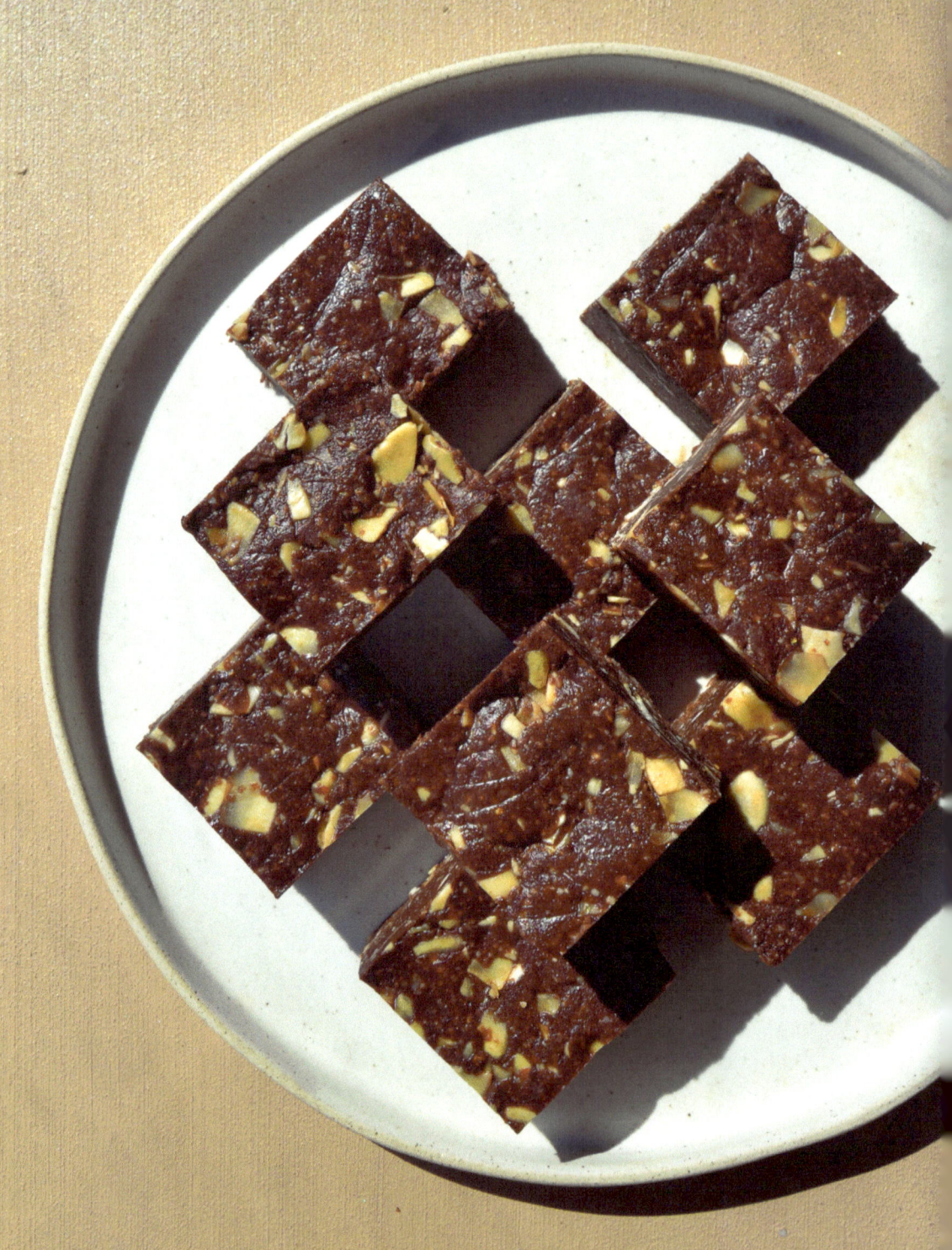

Coconut bacon isn't just for breakfast granola or salad topping anymore. These decadent spicy coconut bacon brownies prove that bacon is just as delicious as dessert!

Time - 30 minutes prepration + 4 hours dehydration + 40 minutes setting
Serves - 9 squares

Spicy Coconut Bacon
40 g thinly peeled fresh coconut slices
15 ml coconut aminos or tamari
1/4 tsp onion powder
1/4 tsp garlic powder
1/4 tsp paprika powder
1/4 tsp licorice salt or pink himalayan salt

Brownie
60 g sprouted oat flour
60 g almond flour
60 g raw cacao powder
40 g coconut sugar powdered
60 g hazelnut butter
80 g maple syrup
30 g coconut oil melted
15 ml coconut aminos or tamari
7.5 ml vanilla extract
40 g dehydrated spicy coconut bacon

SPICY COCONUT BACON
First, start making spicy coconut bacon. Place the thinly sliced coconut in a small bowl.
Add the rest of ingredients and mix well until combined.
Place on a lined dehydrator tray and dehydrate at 42°C for 2 hours then flip onto mesh tray, continue to dehydrate another 2 hours or until completely dried.
Remove from dehydrator, let them cool for 15 minutes. Then they will be ready to use in your recipes. Coconut bacon can be stored in airtight container or mason jars up to 2-3 months.

BROWNIE
Place oat flour, almond flour, cacao powder, coconut sugar and vanilla powder in a food processor. Mix together until well combined.
Then add maple, coconut aminos and melted coconut oil. Process until dough comes together. When you press with your fingers it should be come together easily.
Once done, transfer mixture in a 15×15 cm square cake tin lined parchment paper. Smooth it down with the back of a spoon. Sprinkle dehydrated spicy coconut bacon on the top. Flatten again.
Pop in the freezer to set, about 30-40 minutes. Then cut, slice and serve.

SEMLA

WITH CHOCOLATE AND NUTS

Time - 3 hours prep + 6 hrs dehydration + 1 hour setting
Serves - 9 buns

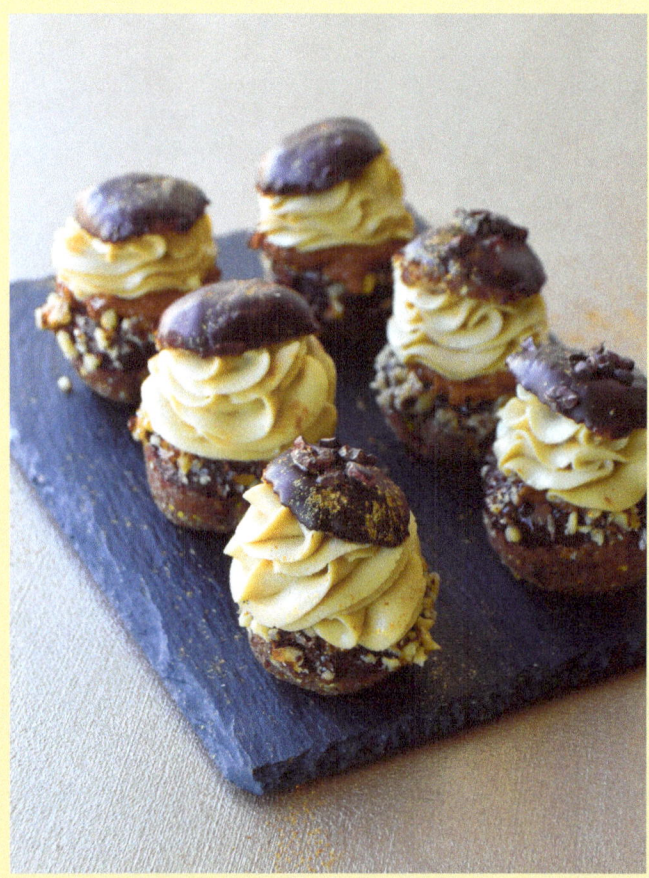
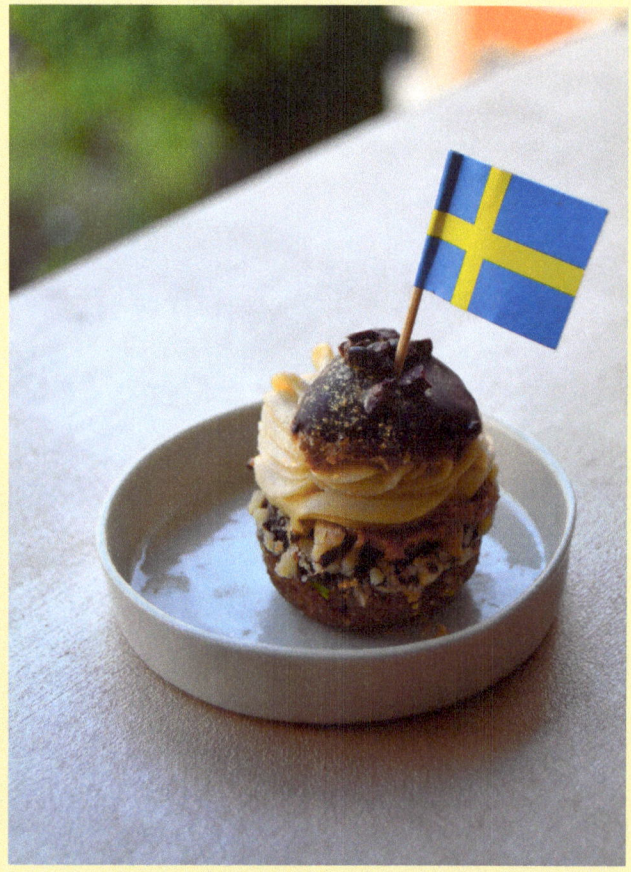

Bun Dough

Dry Ingredients
140 g almond flour
15 g buckini flour or coconut flour
20 g psyllium husk powder
22 g ground flaxseed
4 g cardamom powder
1/2 tsp pink himalayan salt

Wet Ingredients
150 g kohlrabi
75 g medjool dates soaked
15 ml lemon juice

Almond Butter Filling
120 g almond butter
15 ml maple syrup
15 g coconut sugar powdered
4-5 drops almond extract
5 ml vanilla extract
A pinch of licorice salt

White Cream
1 batch white chocolate frosting (page 26)

For Dipping
1 batch raw chocolate melted (page 28)
50 g chopped almonds and raw cacao nibs mixed together

Before you start, make sure you prepared white chocolate frosting beforehand.

BUN DOUGH

To make buns, peel your kohlrabi, cut into small chunks and add to your food processor. Squeeze the lemon over the kohlrabi. Then add the soaked and strained medjool dates. Process until puree.

Add all dry ingredients. Continue to mix the kohlrabi date puree and dry ingredients together until you have a fine dough that sticks together. If the dough feels wet, add 1 tsp buckini flour at a time or if feels dry, add more lemon juice. Knead the dough with your hands and divide between 9 equal pieces. Then roll the pieces into small balls. Put them on your dehydrator tray, press so that they stand firmly and dehydrate in the dehydrator at 42°C for about 6 hours or until you feel that they are a little firm on the outside. They should not be too dry but have a core that is juicy. Carefully cut the top off the buns. Using a small teaspoon or apple core remover, dig the core out a little. Place the lids and buns on the dehydrator sheet, continue to dehydrate for additional 2 hours.

ALMOND BUTTER FILLING

To make almond filling cream, pour the almond butter in a bowl, add the rest of ingredients, whisk well until slightly becomes thicken. Set in the refrigerator during the dehydration process of buns.

ASSEMBLY

Once buns are done, remove them from the dehydrator. Remove the almond cream from the refrigerator. Dip the lid of the dough and the upper part of the bun into the chocolate, then dip the bun into desiccated coconut or chopped almonds so they stick to the chocolate and let it cool quickly in the fridge. Once chocolate is cooled, add 2 tsp almond cream filling in the hollows. Transfer the white cream to a piping bag with preferred tip. Pipe the almond cream starting from the middle of core until achieve a high peak of whipped cream. Put the lid of bun. Enjoy!

RAW FIKA

BLÅBÄRSTÅRTA

SWEDISH BLUEBERRY CAKE

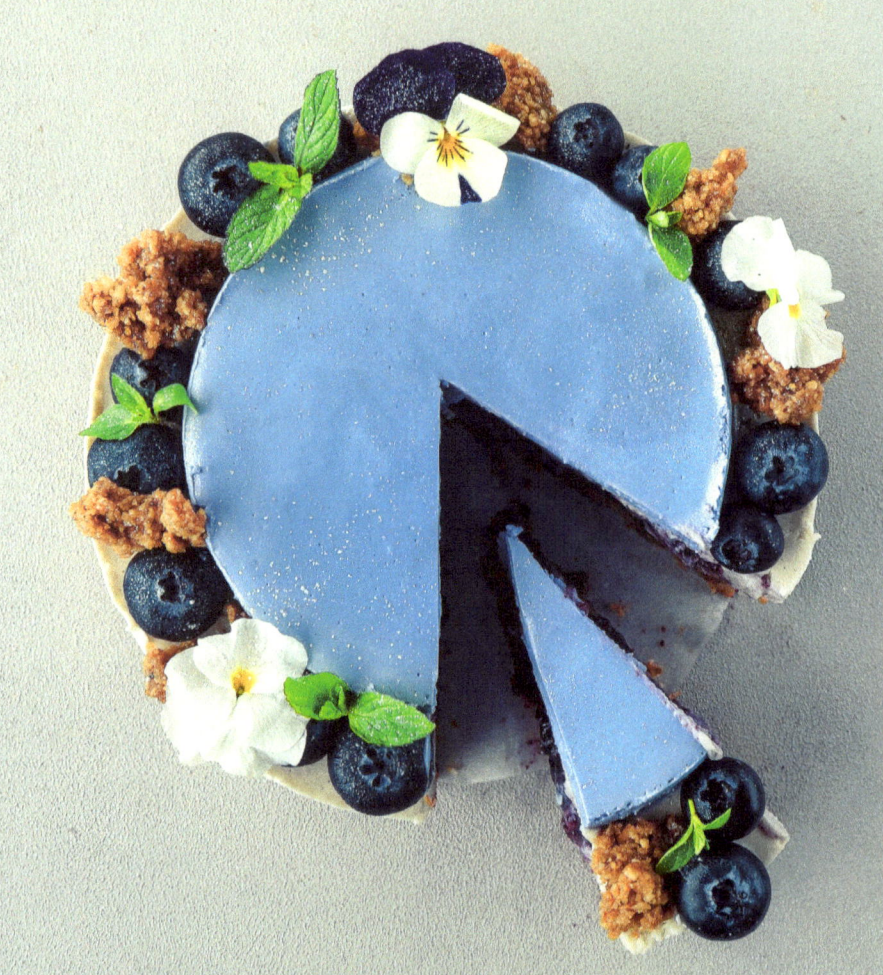

Time - 2 hours + 6-8 hours setting
Serves - 15 cm round cake, 6 slices

Cookie Base
8 g chia seeds
60 ml water
40 g oat flour
10 g coconur flour
50 g walnut
45 g coconut sugar powdered
65 ml maple syrup
60 g hazelnut butter
20 ml virgin coconut oil melted
20 g cacao butter melted

Crust
1 batch cookie dough (page 30, also set aside some pieces for decoration)
10 g cacao butter melted
10 g virgin coconut oil melted
20 ml maple syrup
20 g almond butter
5 g licorice powder (optional)
A good pinch of pink himalayan salt

Blueberry Jam
220 g fresh blueberries
30 ml maple syrup
10 ml lemon juice
5 g chia seeds

Cheesecake Filling
1 batch (130 g) fermented cashew cream (page 29)
100 ml coconut cream
80 ml maple syrup
50 ml virgin coconut oil melted
15 ml cacao butter melted
30 ml lemon juice
5 g nutritional yeast
A pinch pink himalayan salt

Decoration
50 g cookie dough
White pansies
Fresh blueberries
Fresh peppermint

COOKIE BASE

In a mixing bowl, mix chia seeds and water. Keep stirring for the first minute or so to prevent the chia seeds from clumping together. Set aside for 5 minutes.

Then add the rest of ingredients in the chia seed mixture. Stir well to combine.

Transfer the dough onto a baking tray lined parchment paper. Spread with a help of spatula as thin as possible. The shape is not important, we will use it in cake crust later and run into flour. It is just important to spread thinly in order to decrease the dehydration time. Dehydrate for 6-8 hours at 42°C (or overnight) until fully dried.

It can be made beforehand and stored in the airtight container or jar up to 2 months. Once opened the jar, use in the same day.

BLUEBERRY JAM

In the meantime, prepare your blueberry jam the day before as it will take 6 hours. Wash and dry your blueberries, add to a large bowl along with lemon juice, chia seeds and maple. Using a fork, mash your blueberries. Dehydrate for 6 hours or until thick enough.

CRUST

Once your cookie base is ready, set aside few pieces for decoration (appox. 50 g), then transfer rest to a food processor, run into slightly flour, you may have some chunks in it, it is totally fine. Add the rest of crust ingredients. Process until everything combined well. Transfer dough to a 15 cm cake mold lined parchment paper. Press with your hands and then back of a spoon, flatten out as much as possible.

CHEESECAKE FILLING

Meanwhile start making cheesecake filling. Place fermented cashew filling in a high speed blender. Except cacao butter and coconut oil, add all ingredients and blend until everything is well combined and smooth. Lastly add melted cacao butter and coconut oil, process again until silky smooth.

ASSEMBLY

Place a 10 cm round cake mold (without bottom) in the middle of your cake crust. So you have 10 cm mold inside the 15 cm mold now. Pour the blueberry jam into the 10 cm center and flatten it with a teaspoon. Place it in the freezer and leave for 1 hour.

(contintued on the next page)

Once time is up, and the jam is thick enough when you touch with your fingers, remove the crust with jam from the freezer. Unmould the 10 cm cake mold. Do not unmould the 15 cm mold at this stage.
Pour the half cheesecake filling over the crust and blueberry jam. Make sure that the cream is covered the jam layer well.

Gently tap the mold in order to prevent bubbles. Then transfer the cake in the freezer again at least 2 hours.
Add butterfly pea flower pea in the rest of cheesecake filling, blend again until the cream is completely blue and smooth.

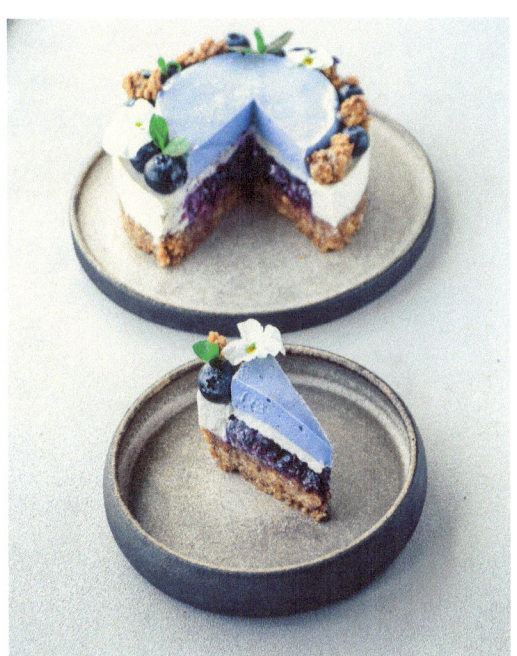

After 2 hours, remove the cake from the freezer. Place the 10 cm cake mold. on the middle of white cheesecake cream.
Pour the blue cheesecake filling in the 10 cm cake mold. Freeze again at least 2-3 hours or completely cooled.

Meanwhile prepare your decoration elements. Wash and dry your blueberries, mint leaves and pansies.

Once time is up, carefully remove 10 cm mold from the blue layer. Then remove the 15 cm mold. Place the cake on a clean plate. Freeze cake again for the next 2 hours. We remove the molds halfway through the freezing process, otherwise it will be difficult when it is completely frozen.
Even if you complete the freezing time, you can leave it outside for a while, so it will be easier to remove the molds. It is important to freeze all the layers evenly to have smooth layers, so I recommend that the cake is free-zed well and then sit in the refrigerator for 2 hours, before cutting.

Instead of using special molds for everything, I mostly prefer to use multi-tiered molds in the form of 5-10-15-20 and its multiples. If you find it easier, you can also use a special mold to make this kind of cakes.

Decorate with rest of your cookie base, fresh mint, blueberries, pansies.

Dust some edible silver powder if desired for a luxury look.

RAW FIKA

KLADDKAKA

SWEDISH STICKY BROWNIE CAKE

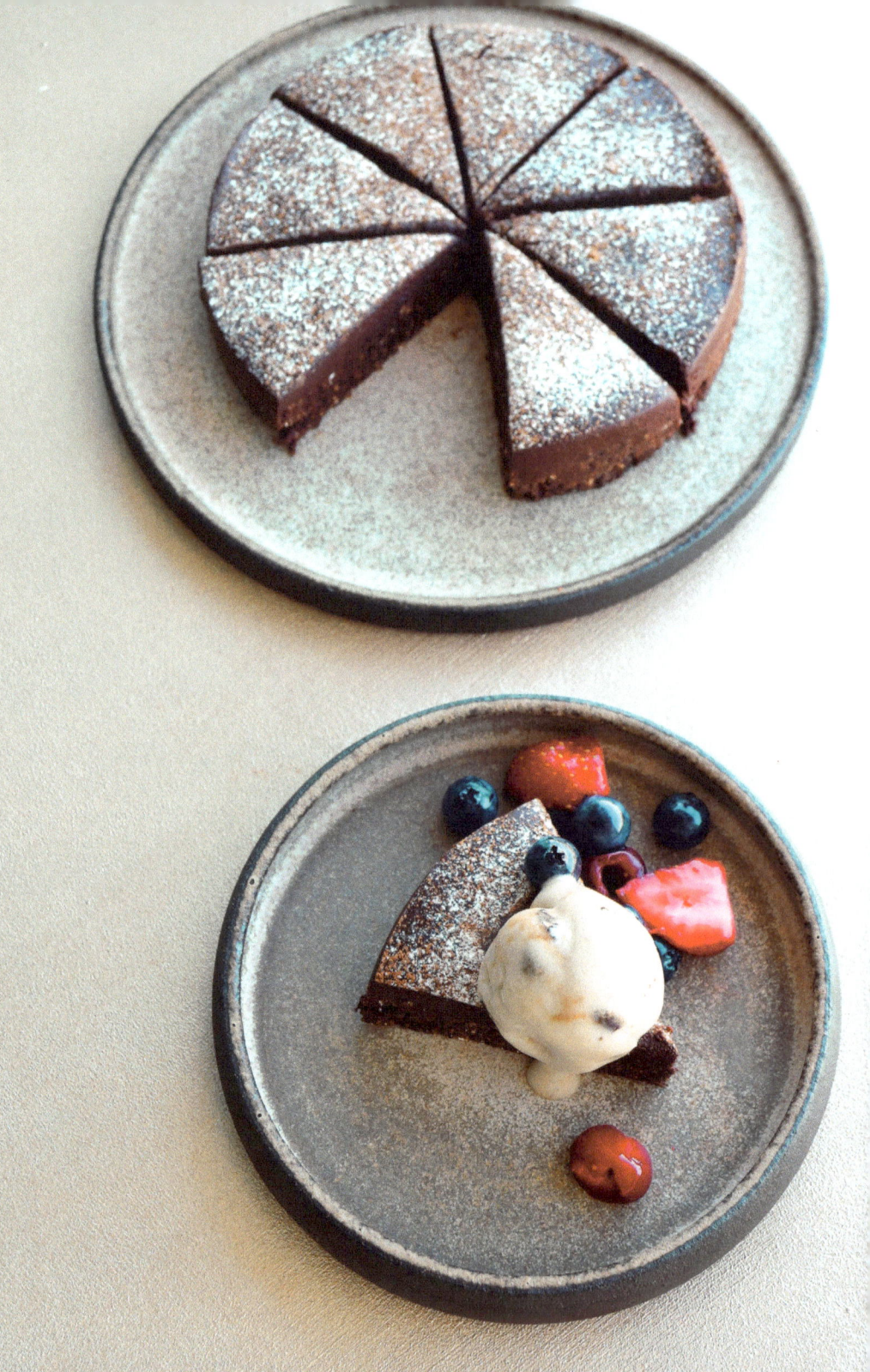

Kladdkaka was actually made by accident. It was baked into existence in 1938 in Örebro, Sweden by Gudrun Isaksson who was originally trying to make brownies with no baking powder. This sugary delicacy, which directly translates to 'mud cake' or 'sticky cake' is definitely a Swedish staple. It is rich and dense, with a delicate, crispy exterior and a soft, gooey centre.. Like many Swedish desserts, it's too easy to make to pass up. Its main ingredients are simply cocoa powder, flour, sugar, and eggs. But can be made healthier, ethical version without animal products. See our new twist with a kick of chunky monkey. The original chunky monkey also includes some walnuts. Our verison is nut-free. But add some walnuts at the end along with the raw cacao nibs if you like. Of course, kladdkaka has its own day of celebration too. Kladdkakans Dag falls on November 7.

Time - 30 minutes prep + 2 hours freezing
Serves - 6

Kladdkaka Dough
85 g oat flour
185 g fresh dates soaked rinsed
35 g raw cacao powder
45 ml coconut milk
1/4 tsp licorice salt

Chunky Monkey Ice Cream
160 g young coconut meat
100 g frozen bananas
100 ml coconut milk
50 ml maple syrup
25 g raw cacao nibs
40 g melted coconut oil
1/4 tsp licorice salt (or pink himalayan salt)
50 g walnuts chopped (optional)

Chocolate Sauce
40 ml virgin coconut oil melted
25 g raw cacao powder
25 g coconut sugar powdered (grind in the coffee grinder beforehand)
75 ml coconut milk
5 ml tamari or coconut aminos

CHUNKY MONKEY ICECREAM
Place the frozen bananas and coconut milk in your high speed blender. Add young coconut meat, maple, melted coconut oil and salt. Let them sit for 5 minutes at room temperature. Then process at ice cream mode. If the consistency is too thick after mixing you can add a splash of coconut milk. Blend until it is the consistency of soft-serve ice cream. Last, add the raw cacao nibs and give a few pulses just to mix in. This will give you a nice crunch in your nice cream. You can also add some chopped walnuts at the end if you want to stick to original chunky monkey. Freeze in an airtight container for 2 hours.

KLADDKAKA DOUGH
Place oat flour, salt and cacao powder in a food processor, mix together. Add dates and coconut milk, process again until you get sticky smooth dough. Place in a 15 cm round cake tin lined parchment paper. Press down the dough, and flatten out as much as possible using a spatula or the back of spoon.

CHOCOLATE SAUCE
Place all chocolate ingredients in a bowl, melt by bain marie method.

ASSEMBLY
Pour the mixture over the cake. Keep in the freezer for 1.5 hours to set. Once the time is up, remove the kladdkaka and ice cream from the freezer. Cut the cake into 6 equal pieces. Scoop a ball from the chunky monkey ice cream. Serve your kladdkaka with icecream and berries if desired.

PRINSESSTÅRTA

SWEDISH PRINCESS CAKE

Time - 4 hours
Serves - 8 cm x 9 pieces round mould

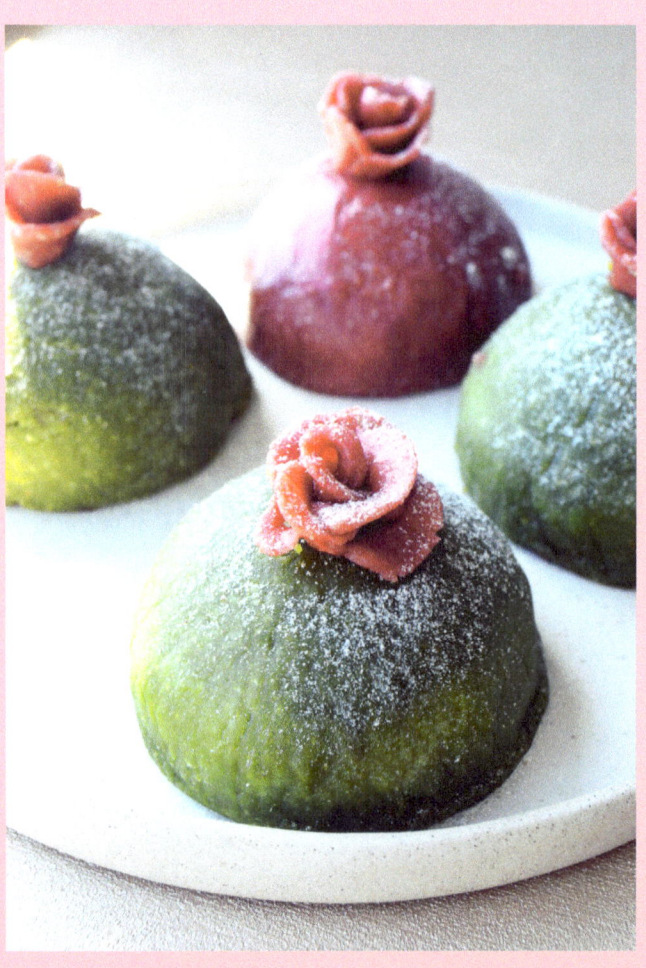
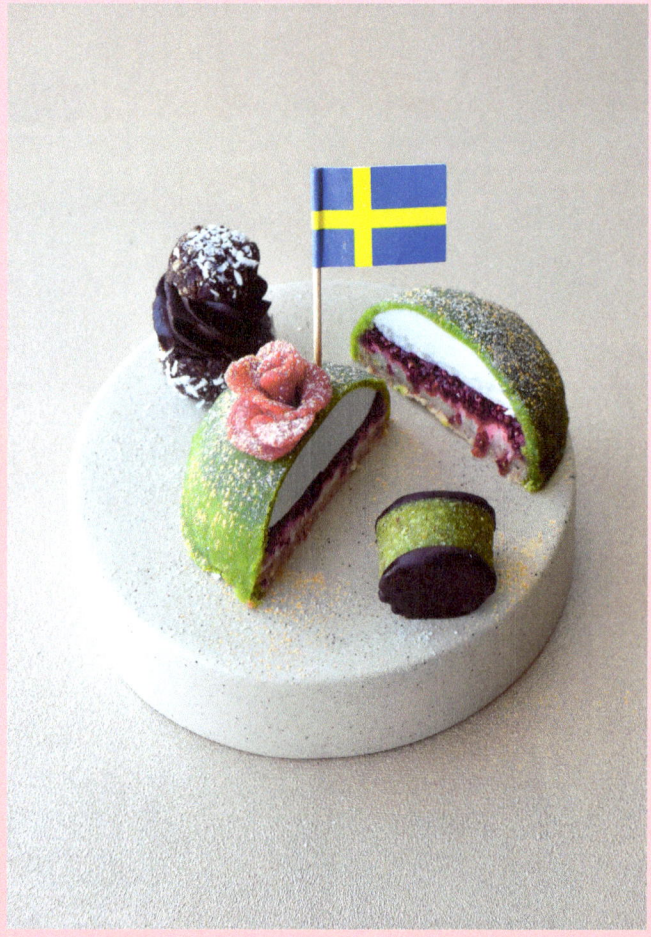

Princess cake is a traditional Swedish layer cake consisting of alternating layers of airy sponge cake, pastry cream, raspberry jam and a thick-domed layer of whipped cream. The cake is covered by a layer of marzipan, giving it a smooth rounded top. The marzipan overlay is usually green, sprinkled with powdered sugar and decorated with a pink marzipan rose.

Our healthy version includes layers of coconut whipped cream, chia berry jam, vanilla custard, almond sponge cake, green marzipan colored with spinach, sprinkled with coconut flour and decorated with strawberry marzipan roses.

This cake requires 8 cm x 9 pieces semi sphere moulds. When finished, turn it with the flat side down on the sponge cake crust and cover it with the green marzipan.

Working with marzipan may take some effort and experience, but a tip to save it from breaking is to keep the syrup ratio high and sit it in the refrigerator for a while to prevent sticking, so you can work easily. Shaping it with slightly wet fingers also will help you!

Coconut Whipped Cream
200 ml coconut cream
60 g irish moss gel
30 g maple syrup
5 ml vanilla extract or vanilla pod powder

Raspberry Chia Jam
250 g raspberries fresh or defrosted
40 ml maple syrup
45 g chia seeds

COCONUT WHIPPED CREAM
Grab a can of chilled coconut cream, discarding the water, if there is any. Add the coconut cream into a medium bowl along with the irish moss gel, maple and vanilla.

With a whisk or electric beater, whip the cream until smooth and fluffy. My tip is to put the bowl and the whisker in the freezer for 10 minutes before whisking, because having the appliances chilled as well will help you avoid melting the cream during the process. Add the 25 g of whipped coconut cream as your first layer in each 8 cm semi sphere mold . Let the mold rest in the freezer while making the strawberry jam.

RASPBERRY CHIA JAM
Just take a fork and mash the defrosted berries, when you only have very small chunks of berries left, add the chia seeds and maple then stir for a minute or two, dehydrate the jam in a bowl for about 45 minutes stirring every 15 minutes or so on. Once the jam is thickened, add 22 g of jam on top of each coconut cream layer. Keep in the freezer. (continutes on the next page)

Vanilla Custard

130 g soaked cashews

55 ml coconut milk

45 ml maple syrup

50 ml virgin coconut oil melted

15 ml lemon juice

5 ml vanilla extract or vanilla pod powder

Sponge Cake Crust

50 g almond flour

50 g rolled oats

30 g coconut flour

40 ml maple syrup

30 g almond butter

15 ml water + more as needed

1/2 tsp cardamom powder

1/2 tsp licorice salt

Green Marzipan

30 g fresh collard greens or spinach

150 g activated dehydrated almond flour

200 ml maple syrup or coconut nectar

40 g raw coconut flour

1/4 tsp spirulina powder

1/8 tsp turmeric powder

VANILLA CUSTARD

Make the cashew vanilla custard by blending all ingredients in a high speed blender and adding the coconut oil at the end. Add a layer of cashew vanilla custard on top of the chia jam layer. Let the cake set in the freezer for at least 2 hours.

SPONGE CAKE CRUST

Make the spongecake layer in a food processor. Roll the dough between two parchment paper. Flatten and cut with a 8 cm round cutter into 9 pieces.

Make sure your cakes frozen all the way through. Once ready, flip the cakes upside down on the sponge cake crusts.

GREEN MARZIPAN

To make the green marzipan, start by blending the maple, spinach, spirulina and turmeric in a high speed blender until you have a smooth green sauce. Then using a strainer, strain the mixture, remove the pulp. Transfer the syrup into a bowl, add the almond flour and work the dough with your hands while adding the coconut flour until you get a very firm dough with marzipan texture. When it's done, let it sit in the fridge for 15 minutes.

Transfer the marzipan between two baking paper, roll the dough flat with a rolling pin. Carefully place the green marzipan on the cake. Cut the edges and make it look as smooth as possible. Knead the edges and roll the marzipan again. Repeat the process for the rest of cakes.

When the cakes are done, dust with some coconut flour, put strawberry marzipan rose on the top of each cake.

(continutes on the next page)

Strawberry Marzipan Roses

50 g activated dehydrated almond flour

30 g freeze dried strawberry or raspberry powder

25 ml maple syrup or coconut nectar syrup

3 g filtered water

2 g freshly squeezed lemon juice

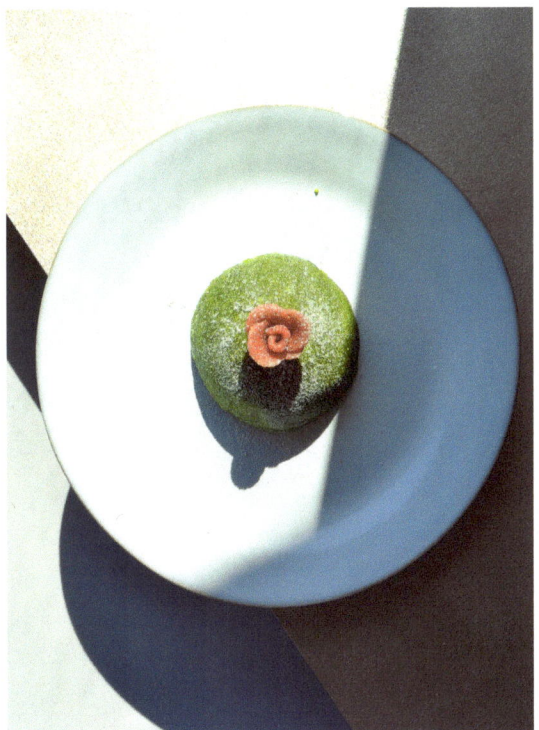

STRAWBERRY MARZIPAN ROSES

Place almond flour and freeze dried strawberry powder in a food processor, mix together.
Then add maple syrup, water and lemon juice, blend together. After a few pulses, the marzipan comes together.

Roll the marzpian into a ball and flatten it between two parchment paper. Refrigerate for 2 hours before sharping in order to prevent sticking.

Remove from the freezer, using a 2,5 cm small round cutter, cut the dough into 54 small 2,5 cm marzipan rounds.

You will make 9 marzipan roses for each cake and will need 6 small rounds for each rose.

Once cut the marzpian into 2,5 cm rounds, gently press down the edges using your fingers to make nice delicate edges.
Take one petal and roll it between your fingers to create the center bud.

Add petals around the bud, overlapping at times. Remember nature isn't perfect and these don't need to be either. Don't worry about the chunky back. Focus on making a nice flower first.
Once you are happy with the front, gently slice off the excess on the back.
Roll it enough to smooth it out, but keep the back flat so it can sit up straight. These roses will keep for days. You can cover in plastic wrap or let the air make a slight crust.

RAW FIKA RECIPES

RAW FIKA

SCHACKRUTOR
SWEDISH CHESSBOARD COOKIES

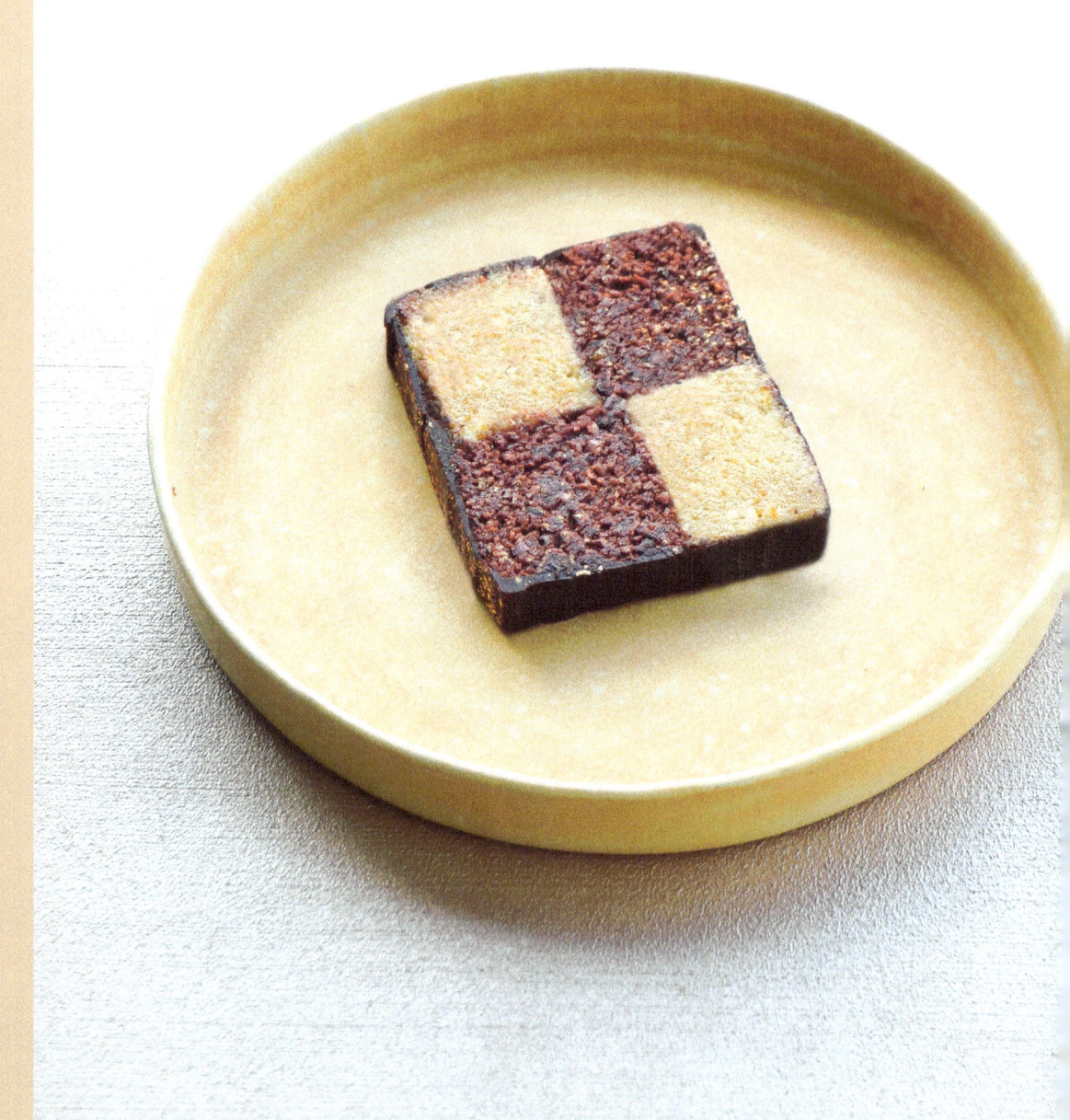

These chessboard cookies are perfect for when you can't decide if you want a chocolate or vanilla cookie! This is an easy cookie recipe that looks impressive, but is simple and fun to make!

2×2 size is the most common, you can also make 4x4 or whatever you like. We made 4x4 size here. A thin rim in one of the colors is also a popular tweak, we prefer our raw version with chocolate covered edge. If you end up having any leftovers of the dough, squeeze them together to a mixed roll and cut them into coins.

Time - 40 min prep + 3 hours setting
Serves - 8-10

Chocolate Dough

80 g medjool dates (weight after pitted)
50 ml maple syrup
10 g raw cacao nibs
76 g almond flour
60 g rolled oat flour
20 g shredded coconut
30 g raw cacao powder
15 ml freshly brewed espresso
A pinch pink himalayan salt
22 g virgin coconut oil melted

Vanilla Dough

135 g almond flour or cashew flour
15 g coconut flour
90 ml maple syrup
15 ml virgin coconut oil melted
A pinch pink himalayan salt
5 ml vanilla extract
1 orange zest

Chocolate Dipping

100 g raw chocolate melted

CHOCOLATE DOUGH

Place the oat flour, almond flour, shredded coconut, salt and raw cacao powder in your food processor. Mix together. Then add the medjool dates, maple syrup, espresso and melted coconut oil. Process until dough comes together. Lastly add the raw cacao nibs and process again.

Divide the dough into two equal halves. For a 4x4 cookie, divide each dough balls into two. Form each ball into a square-shaped long bar, about 2 cm thick and high. Wrap and chill the log for 2-3 hours so it firms up and is easier to cut.

VANILLA DOUGH

Place the almond flour, coconut flour and salt into the food processor. Mix together. Then add the maple syrup, coconut oil, vanilla extract and orange zest. Process until dough holds together. Wrap and chill the log for at least 2-3 hours or longer until firm enough.

ASSEMBLY

Place one dark log next to a white and gently squeeze them together. Add the two remaining logs on top so they form a checkerboard pattern. Squeeze gently but try to keep the square shape of the logs. You can dab them with a little bit of coconut oil if it is difficult to make them stick together, but that usually isn't necessary. Wrap and freeze the dough again at least 40-50 minutes. Once done, dip in the melted raw chocolate. Place in a parchment paper and chill until the chocolate rim is thicken. Then cut and serve. Store in the refrigerator up to a week.

CHOKLADBOLLAR

RAW FIKA

SWEDISH CHOCOLATE BALLS

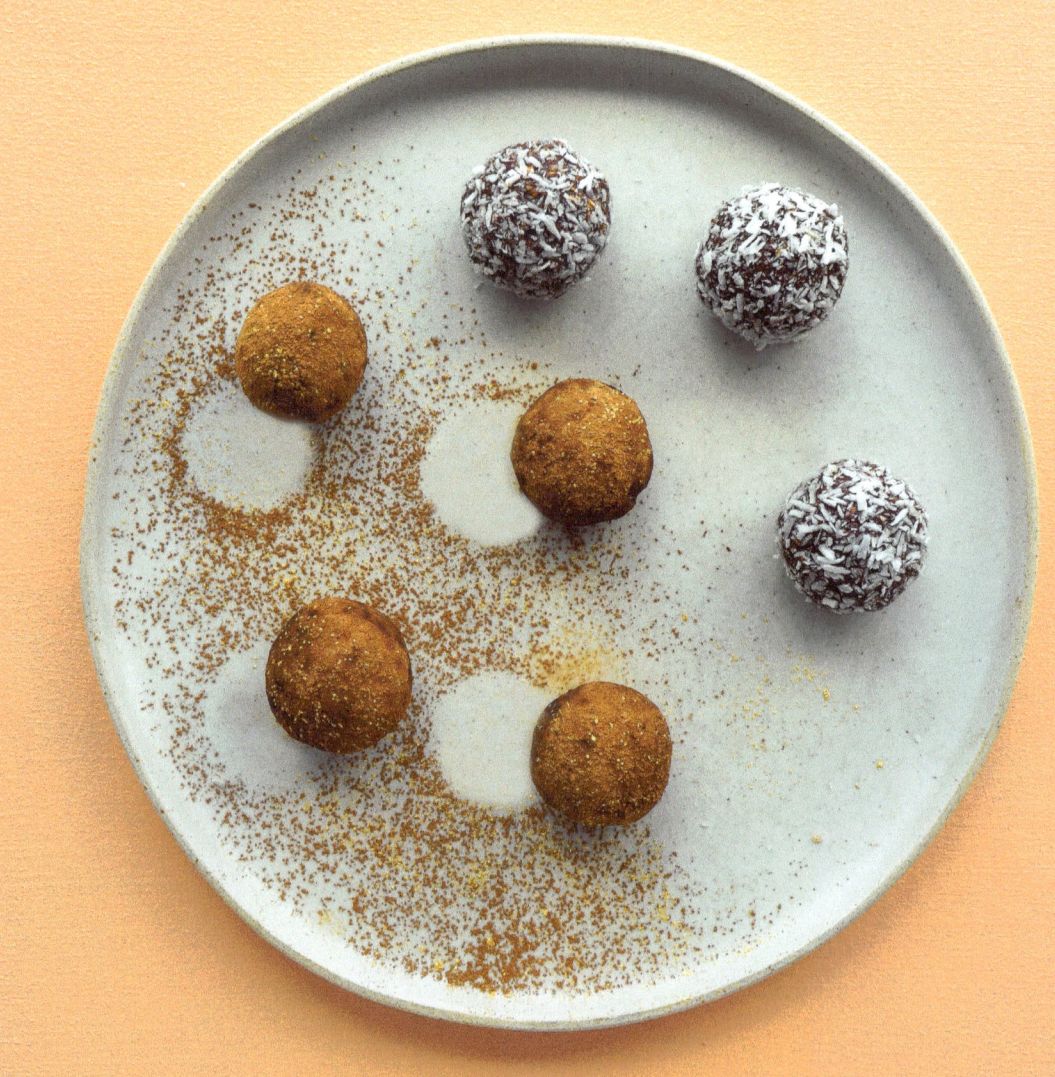

Chokladbollar is one of the simplest sweets to make . You don't even need to bake them – just pop them in the fridge! They were introduced in Sweden in 1943 and were a way to use up leftover ingredients during times of scarcity. Swedes celebrate this pastry on Chokladbollens Dag or Chocolate Ball Day every year on May 11.

Traditionally in Sweden, chokladbollar consist of oats, butter, refined sugar and cocoa, delicious but not the sort of treat you can eat every day. What makes raw version nourishing is that the quality of cacao and coconut of course. In addition the sweetener. These ingredients give this delicious treat a luxurious, indulgent texture; simple larder ingredients that you almost always have to hand too.
A soft, strong hit of chocolate, in its most intense form. You'll certainly love this recipe!

Ingredients

120 g gluten-free rolled oats
40 g desiccated coconut
30 g almond butter
15 ml virgin coconut oil melted
45 g raw chocolate melted
30 g coconut sugar
7 g raw cacao powder
4 tbsp freshly brewed espresso
7 ml tamari or 15 ml coconut aminos
A pinch of pink himalayan salt

30 g desiccated coconut for coating
or raw cacao powder blended with edible gold powder

INSTRUCTIONS

Melt the raw chocolate and coconut oil together using bain marie method.
Meanwhile, put the rolled oats and coconut sugar in a high speed blender. Process until combined and almost in powder form.
Then add the raw cacao powder and salt, blend to combine together.
Pour the melted raw chocolate, coconut oil, almond butter, coconut aminos and coffee over the mixture. Mix everything until the dough perfectly holds together. You'll see big ball in the food processor when it starts to get a dough shape.
Then remove from the food processor. Make 12 balls with your hands.
Roll in the desiccated coconut or raw cacao powder.

TIPS

-Use best possible ingredients! There aren't many ingredients in chokladbollar so your oats, cacao powder, coconut and coffee should be of good quality. The cacao powder should be a raw to get that pure intense taste.
-Crumble your oats. When selecting oats, I like to use sprouted rolled oats and they should be crumbled after pouring them into the mixing bowl by hand or in a food processor.
-I like to use coconut sugar instead of liquid sweetener because it makes a slightly caramelized taste to the chocolate balls.

RAW FIKA

PEPPARKAKSBOLLAR

SWEDISH GINGERBREAD BALLS

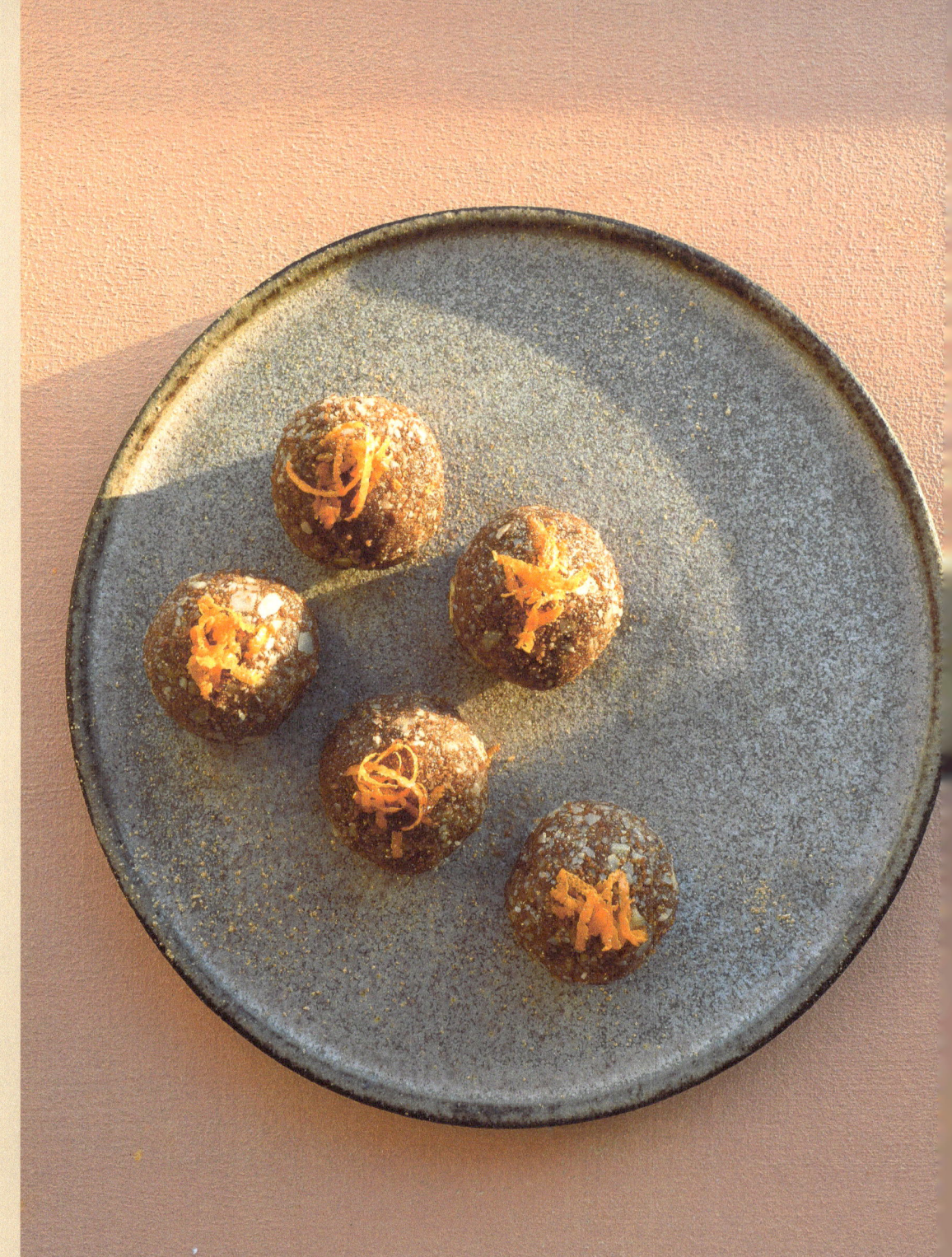

Spicy with aromas of cinnamon, ginger, clove, cardamom and other spices, pepparkakor - the Swedish version of gingerbread, also known as "pepperkake" in Norway, and "piparkakku" in Finland, has the taste of Scandinavian Christmas.

In our raw version, used wild orange essential oil as well and blended with candided almonds. With this high-end rich flavor, it will definitely be one of your future Christmas fika favourites.

Time - 20 min prep + 6 hrs dehydration
Serves - 10-12 balls

Candided Almonds
100 g almonds
45 g coconut sugar
5-6 drops orange essential oil
10 g grated fresh ginger
15 ml fresh ginger juice
20 g raw cacao nibs

Balls
1 batch candided almonds
90 g almond butter
50 g dates soaked
40 ml virgin coconut oil melted
1/2 tsp cinnamon powder
1/8 tsp nutmeg
1/4 tsp licorice

Topping
2 Orange zest

INSTRUCTIONS
Rinse your almonds well and strain.

Then place the almonds, coconut sugar, fresh ginger, ginger juice, raw cacao nibs and orange essential oil in a food processor fitted with an S blade and process until you get a chunky texture.
Place on a dehydrator tray lined parchment or silicon paper and dehydrate at 42°C overnight until completely dried.

Once done, remove from dehydrator, place in a bowl and sit in fridge for 20-30 minutes. This will provide optimal crunch and cool them.

Once cooled enough, process in the food processor fitted with an S blade until a small chunky texture is achieved.

Then add nutmeg, salt, cinnamon powder, soaked rinsed dates, almond butter and melted coconut oil. Process to combine together. Add 1-2 tbsp water if needed to achieve the smooth texture. Make bliss balls from the dough. Keep in the fridge up to a week.

RAW FIKA

HALLONGROTTOR

SOFT RASPBERRY CAVES

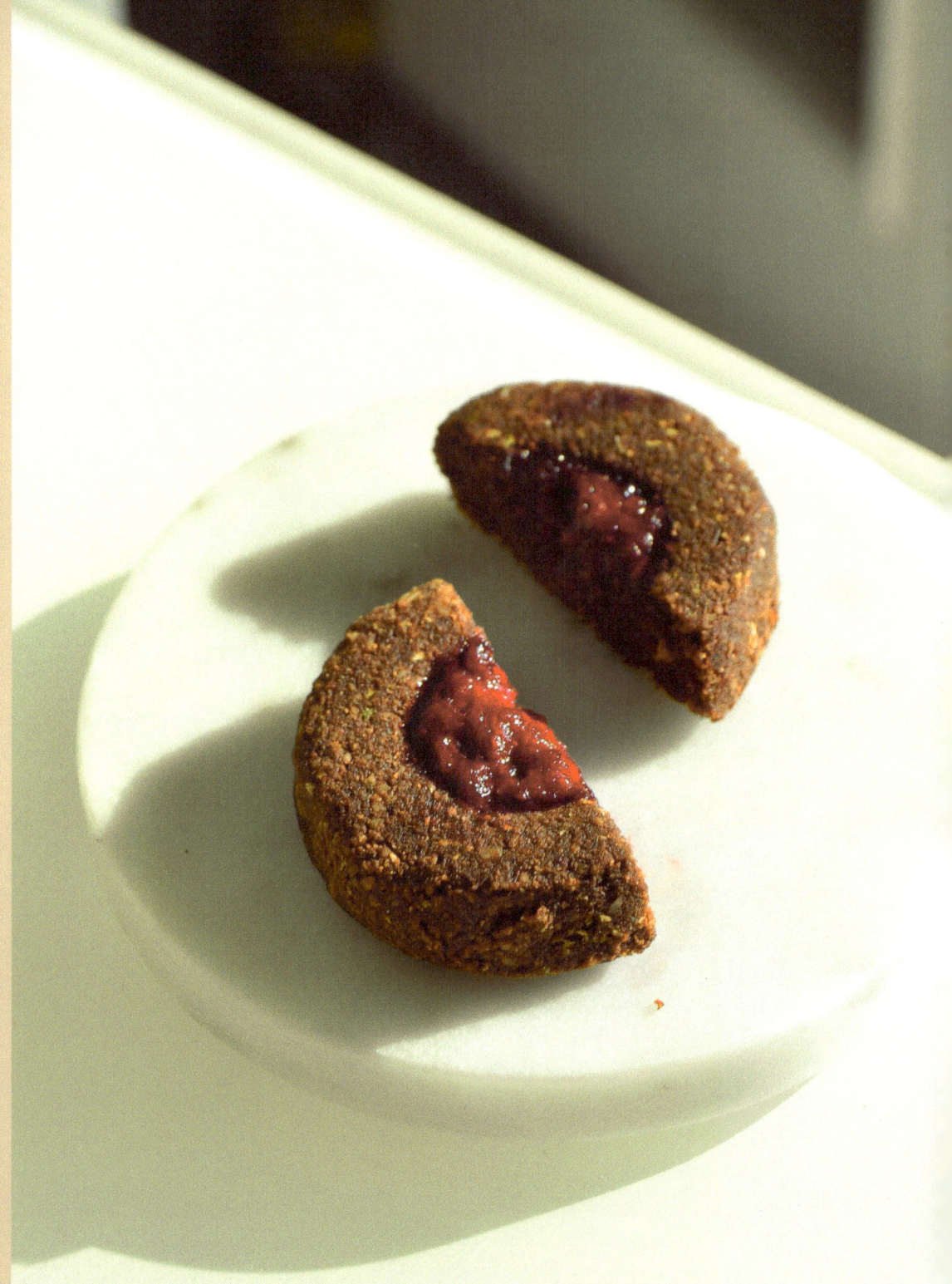

Raspberry caves with sweet raspberry jam and shortcrust pastry. A popular and classic sweet that melts in your mouth. In Sweden, these small cookies are often served to accompany coffee, tea or other hot drinks. Hallongrotta, or hallangrottor in the plural form, means "raspberry cave" in Swedish.

Time - 2 hours prep + 6 hrs dehydration
Serves - 18-20

Dough
Dry Ingredients
140 g almond flour
20 g coconut flour
80 g coconut sugar
25 g psyllium husk powder
20 g ground flaxseed
30 g raw cacao powder
1/2 tsp pink himalayan salt

Wet Ingredients
200 g zucchini
15 ml virgin coconut oil melted
30 ml lemon juice

Raspberry Filling
300 g defrosted raspberries or cherries
10 g chia seeds
15 g coconut sugar
15 ml lemon juice

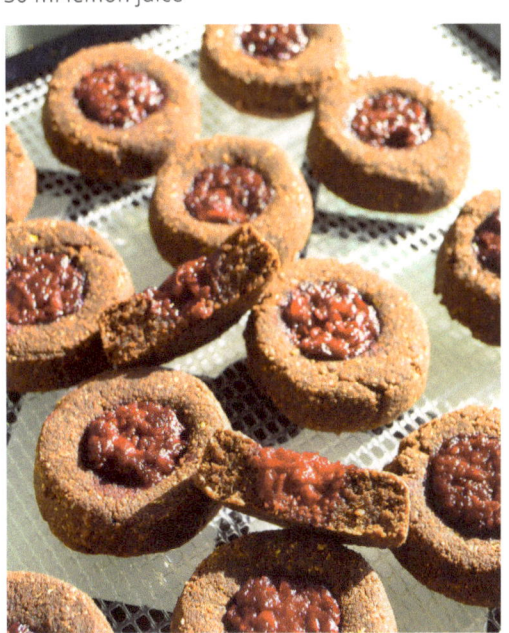

DOUGH
Peel your zucchini, cut into small chunks and add to your food processor. Squeeze the lemon over the zucchini. Then add the coconut sugar. Process until puree. Add all dry ingredients. Continue to mix the zucchini mixture and dry ingredients together until you have a fine dough that sticks together. If the dough feels wet, add 1 tsp coconut flour at a time or if feels dry, add more lemon juice. Knead the dough with your hands and divide between 18-20 equal pieces. Then roll the pieces into small balls. Make a fairly deep 'cave' with your finger in each ball. Put them on your dehydrator tray, press so that they stand firmly and dehydrate in the dehydrator at 42 degrees for about 6 hours or until you feel that they are a little firm on the outside. They should not be too dry but have a core that is juicy.

RASPBERRY FILLING
To make raspberry filling, place all ingredients except chia in a blender, puree them. Then add the chia seeds and stir well. Dehydrate for 5-6 hours or until you achieve desired thick consistency.

ASSEMBLY
After 4 hours of dehydration, fill the holes with raspberry jam. Dehydrate another 2 hours.
They can be eaten immediately or stored in an airtight container up to 4-5 days.

RAW FIKA

RULLTÅRTA

BLACK FOREST ROLL CAKE

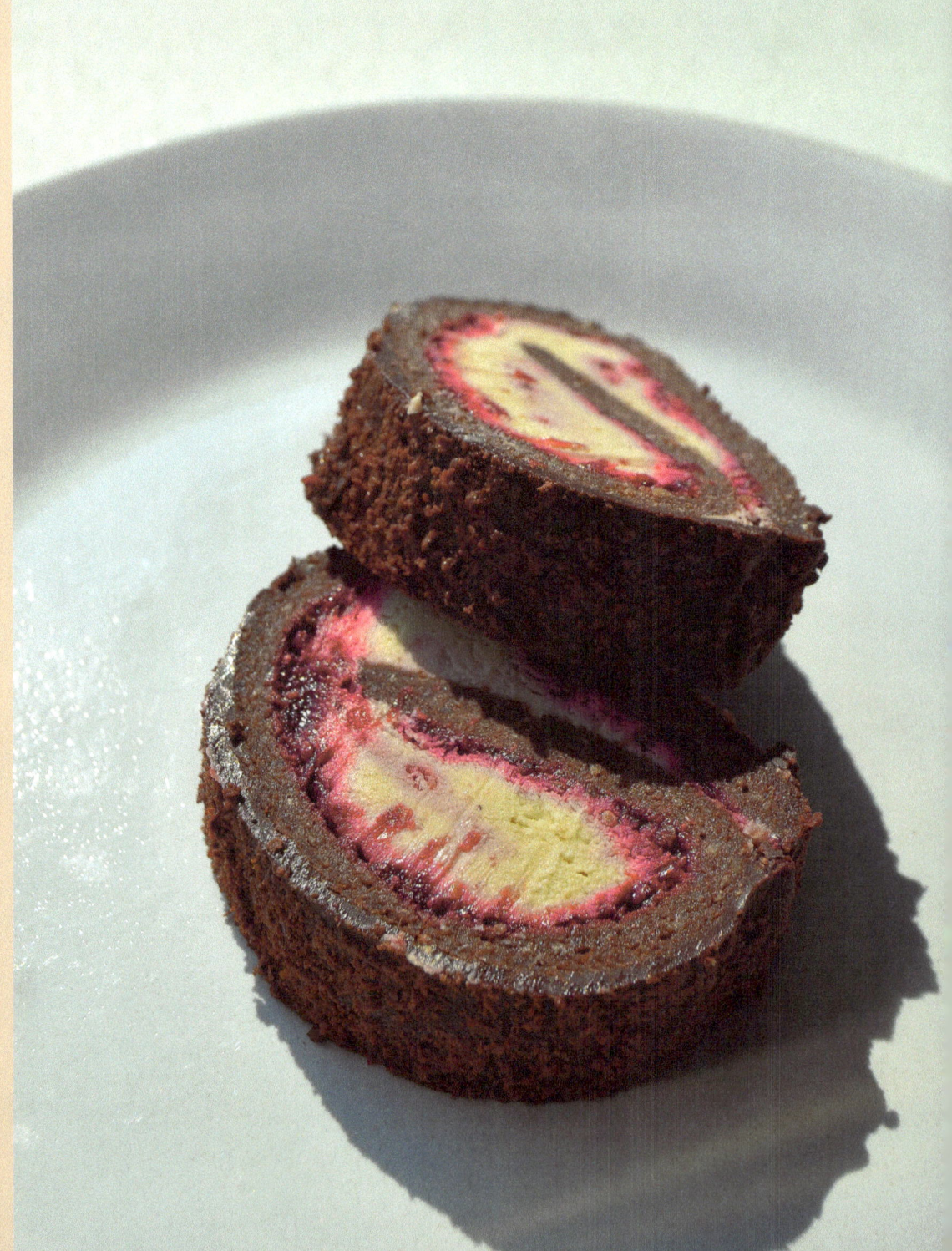

Although Swiss roll is not Swedish, it still gets its own day in Sweden on the 9th of August. Rulltårta comes in many forms and varieties but the two most common are the vanilla sponge with jam filling and the chocolate sponge with buttercream and jam inside. In our raw version, the dehydrated raw pastry is moist and spongy. The jam is a perfect balance of sweet and tangy with sour cherries. And the sweet buttercream is made with nuts.

Time - 1 hour prep + 8 hrs dehydration
Serves - 10

Dehydrated Pastry
275 g kohlrabi
500 ml water
55 ml maple syrup
40 ml sesame oil (or olive oil)
40 g coconut sugar
45 g oat flour
40 g raw cacao powder
90 g almond flour
30 g coconut flour
25 g psyllium husk powder
1/4 tsp salt

Pine Buttercream
140 g pine nuts (or young coconut meat, cashews, macadamia) soaked
130 ml almond milk
60 g maple syrup
40 ml lemon juice
45 g raw cacao butter melted
5 ml vanilla extract

Jam
1 batch lingonberry or sour cherry jam (page 29)

Chocolate Layer
150 g melted raw chocolate (page 28)
50 g shredded raw chocolate (page 28) or use packaged one

DEHYDRATED PASTRY DOUGH

Peel your kohlrabi cut into chunks, add to your blender. Then add the water, oil, salt and maple syrup. Blend until smooth. Set aside.

Meanwhile, add the dry ingredients in a food processor. Blend the flours, cacao, psyllium, salt and sugar together. Pour the kohlrabi batter from the blender over the flour mix. Process until everything combines well. Let it sit for 5 minutes so psyllium absorbs the water content and you get a slightly thick mixture. Divide the mixture in two. You will need two 15x15 cm dehydrator sheet for this. Spread the mixture on nonstick dehydrator trays. Trim the edges nice and neat. Dehydrate for 2 hours, then flip the dough using another dehydrator sheet. Continue to dehydrate for another 6 hours. You might need to flip every 2 hours or so on during the dehydration process.

PINE CREAM

Place all pine cream ingredients except cacao butter in the blender. Blend until silky smooth. Lastly add the melted cacao butter. Blend again to combine together. Freeze the mixture for 2 hours or until thick enough to spread.

ASSEMBLY

Make the jam according to instructions on the page 29.

Spread the jam on the dehydrated pastry nicely. Then pop it back in the dehydrator for 20-30 minutes to dry and firm up a little more. Once done remove from the dehydrator and place in the freezer for 20-30 minutes. This makes it easier to spread the pine cream.

Remove the pine cream from the freezer. Warm it in the dehydrator for a little while. That will loosen it up. Do not overheat or you may lose the emulsification and the oils will separate. Then spread over the jam layer.

Using parchment under the pastry carefully lift up the edge and start to roll. This helps avoid cracking of the pastry. Transfer the roll on a cooling tray. Pour the melted chocolate over the roll, make sure coated all the parts of the roll.

Sprinkle shredded raw chocolate over the roll. Place in the freezer for an hour or so, then you will be able to cut it cleanly.

RAW FIKA

LUSSEKATTER
SWEDISH LUCIA BUNS

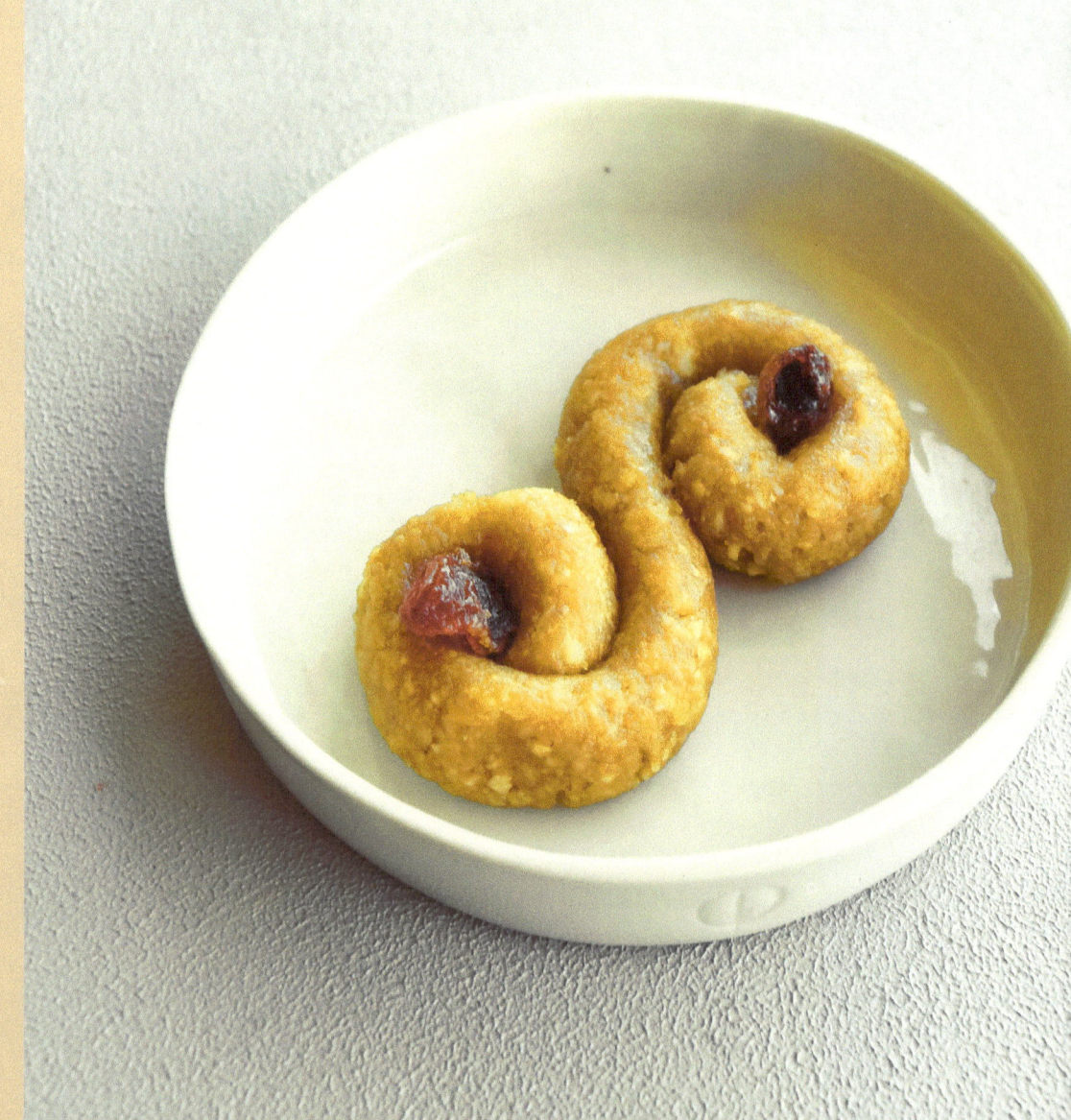

In mid-December, on the shortest day in the medieval Julian calendar, Swedes get up early to celebrate Saint Lucy's Day - December 13th (Luciadag).

Saint Lucia, known in English as Saint Lucy, was a Sicilian saint who became a Christian martyr when she refused to denounce her faith, despite being tortured and set on fire. Swedes across the country commemorate this day with a candlelit procession and eat sweet saffron buns called lussekatter, ginger snaps and mulled wine (glögg). In this recipe, saffron is an essential ingredient which gives the buns yellow colour and a distinctive taste.

Time - 20 min prep + 1 hour setting
Serves - 15 pieces

Ingredients

100 g almond flour
40 g oat flour
75 g cashew flour
20 g coconut flour
15 g desiccated coconut
5 g psyllium husk powder
1/4 tsp saffron +1.5 warm water (dissolve saffron in water) we will use it with both the flowers and water in the dough mixture once dissolved
100 ml maple syrup
20 ml virgin coconut oil melted (use at room temperature or melt using bain marie method)
A pinch of pink himalayan salt

Garnish

15 dried raisins

INSTRUCTIONS

Mix all the ingredients together into a dough.
Make a ball the dough, cover with plastic wrap. Keep in the freezer for 15-20 minutes.
Divide the dough 15 equal pieces.
Roll each pieces and shape into small louse cats.
Garnish with raisins.
Store in a refrigerator or freezer.

CHOCOLATE ORANGE SQUARES

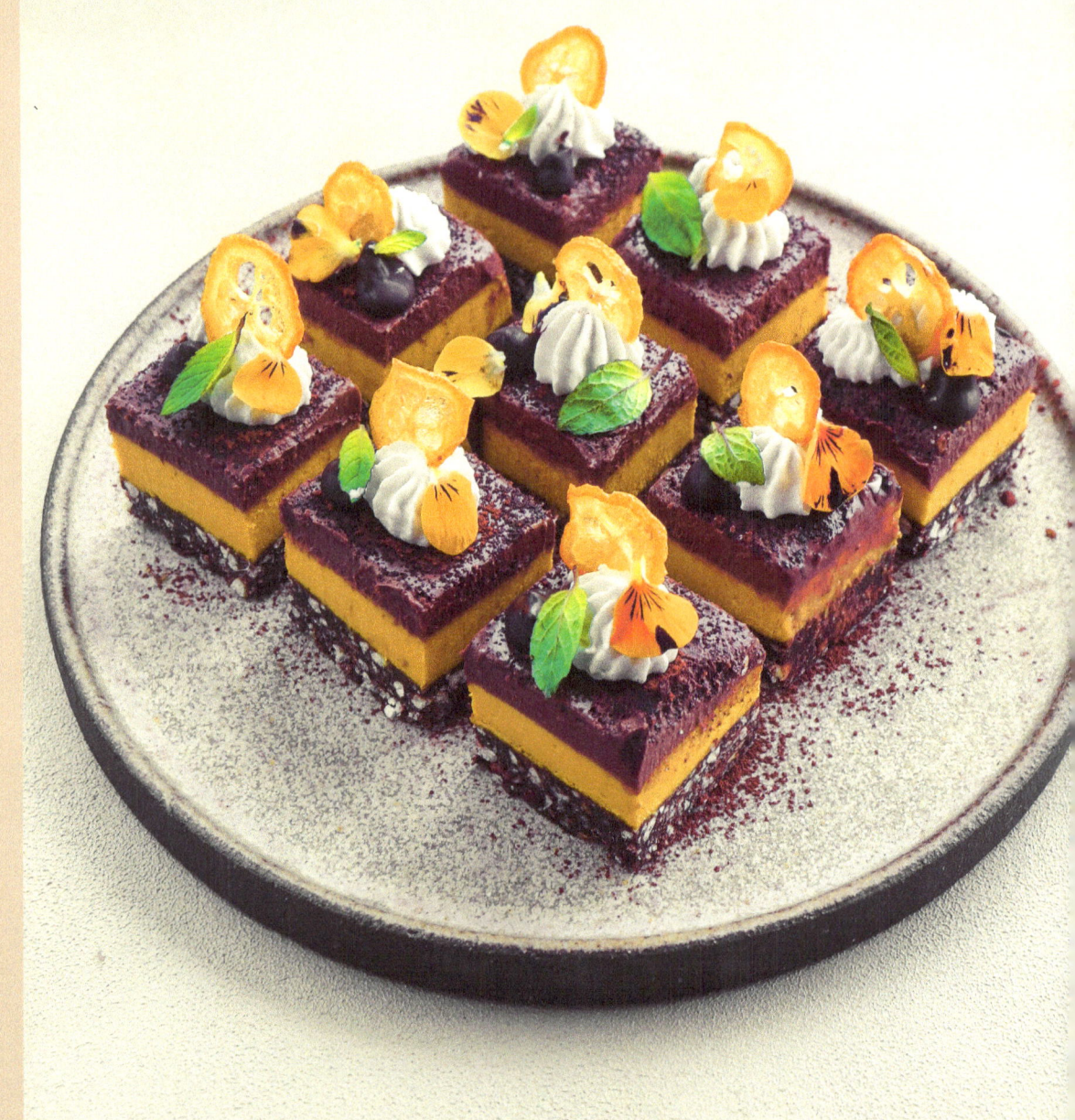

Time - 1 hour + 4 hour setting
Serves - 9

Crust
40 g almond flour
20 g desiccated coconut
25 g coconut flour
15 g raw cacao powder
10 ml tamari
40 ml maple syrup
30 ml virgin coconut oil melted
5 g flaxseeds
65 g buckini

Orange Cream
75 g raw cashews soaked
40 ml kumquat juice (or other citrus)
45 ml coconut cream
45 ml coconut nectar syrup
10 g gojiberry soaked
4-5 drops orange essential oil
10 g raw cacao butter melted
20 g coconut oil melted

Chocolate Ganache
50 g raw cacao butter melted
40 ml maple syrup
35 ml coconut cream
40 ml coconut milk
10 g raw cacao powder
5 ml vanilla extract
4 drops orange essential oil

Decoration
200 g coconut whipped cream
50 g melted raw chocolate
Dehydrated kumquats
Pansies and mint to decorate

CRUST
In a food processor, process the almond flour, desiccated coconut, coconut flour, raw cacao powder and flaxseeds together.
Add the tamari, maple syrup, coconur oil and buckini and process a few times until combined.
Line a 15x15 cm square mold with parchment paper and press the dough evenly. Place into the freezer for 30 min until it firms up.

ORANGE CREAM
To prepare orange cream filling, rinse the cashews and drain them well. Blend all ingredients together (except coconut oil and cacao butter) in a high-speed blender until you reach a nice and smooth consistency. Stream in melted coconut oil and cacao butter and blend until incorporated.

CHOCOLATE GANACHE
To make chocolate ganache, place all ingredients in a small high speed blender and process until smooth. (Blendtec blender with Twister jar works great here.) The important thing is that coconut cream and coconut milk should be at room temperature, otherwise when you mixed them, cold coconut cream can solidify the cacao butter very quickly and prevent it from spilling and fragmentation in between.

ASSEMBLY
Pour orange cream filling over the crust and freeze for at least 2 hours. Just touch with your finger to check its firmness, so when you pour the chocolate ganache over the orange cream, they will not be mixed. Once orange cream is set, remove from the freezer. Pour the chocolate ganache on top. Freeze for at least 3-4 hours.
Meanwhile transfer whipped coconut cream in a piping bag with Wilton 4B noozle. In another piping bag without noozle, pour melted raw chocolate in it. Remove the cake from the freezer. Cut into 9 equal squares.
Pipe the coconut whipped cream and then drop melted chocolate. Decorate with dehydrated kumquats, yellow and orange pansies, fresh mint.

RAW FIKA

TIRAMISU
THE SWEDISH WAY

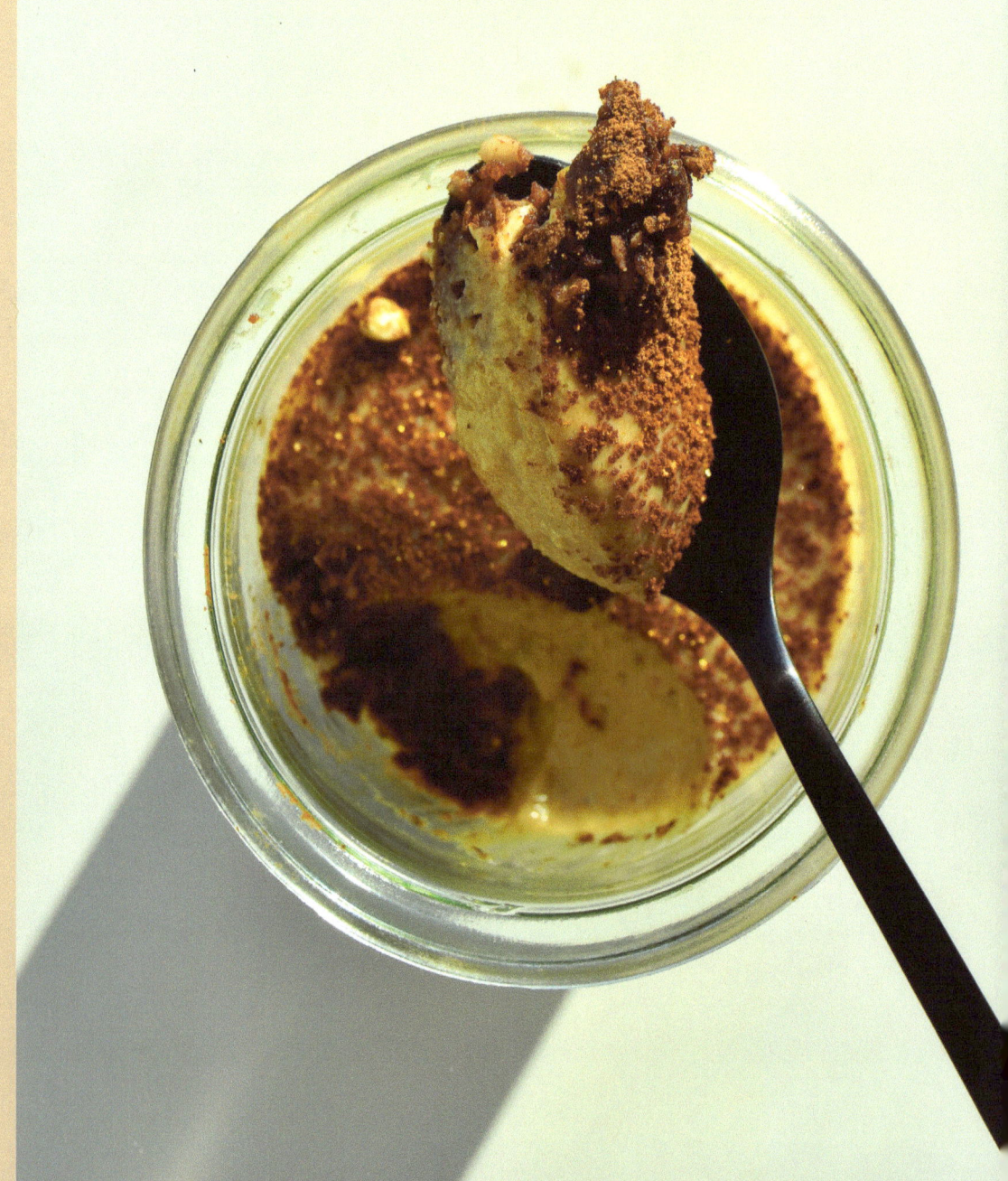

Tiramisu the Swedish way is much healthier, full of fiber and plant-based proteins from oats.

Time - 30 min prep + 1 hour setting
Serves - 160 ml x 4 small weck jars

Kladdkaka Crust
40 g sprouted oat flour
20 g desiccated coconut
70 g medjool dates pitted
15 g hazelnut butter or coconut oil
10 g buckini (sprouted dehydrated buckwheat groats)
10 g raw cacao powder
1/8 tsp cinnamon powder
A pinch of licorice salt
A pinch of nutmeg

Oat Mascarpone
65 g rolled sprouted oats
95 g coconut cream
70 ml coconut milk
20 ml cold press coffee
50 g medjool dates pitted
30 ml maple syrup
20 g hazelnut butter or coconut oil
1/4 tsp cinnamon powder

To serve
Raw cacao powder
Coffee beans

OAT MASCARPONE
To make oat mascarpone, place the oats in a bowl, add the coconut milk. Let it sit for at least 30 minutes or overnight.

Then transfer to your blender, add the coconut cream, cold press coffee, maple, medjool dates and cinnamon. Blend until silky smooth. Lastly add the hazelnut butter or coconut oil. Blend again until everything combined well and you get a smooth mixture.

KLADDKAKA CRUST
To make the kladdkaka crust, place the oats, desiccated coconut, buckini, cinnamon and salt in food processor, blend together.
Then add the medjool dates and hazelnut butter. Combine together. If you need, add a tbsp water. The dough should come together when you press with your hands.

ASSEMBLY
Transfer the mixture between jars. Pour the cream over the crusts. The recipes makes 4 small weck jars (160 ml)

Dust some raw cacao and drop coffee beans. Let it sit in the refrigerator for 4-5 hours or overnight. Serve cold.

RAW FIKA

TRUFFLE HELIODOR

GIFT OF THE SUN TO THE EARTH

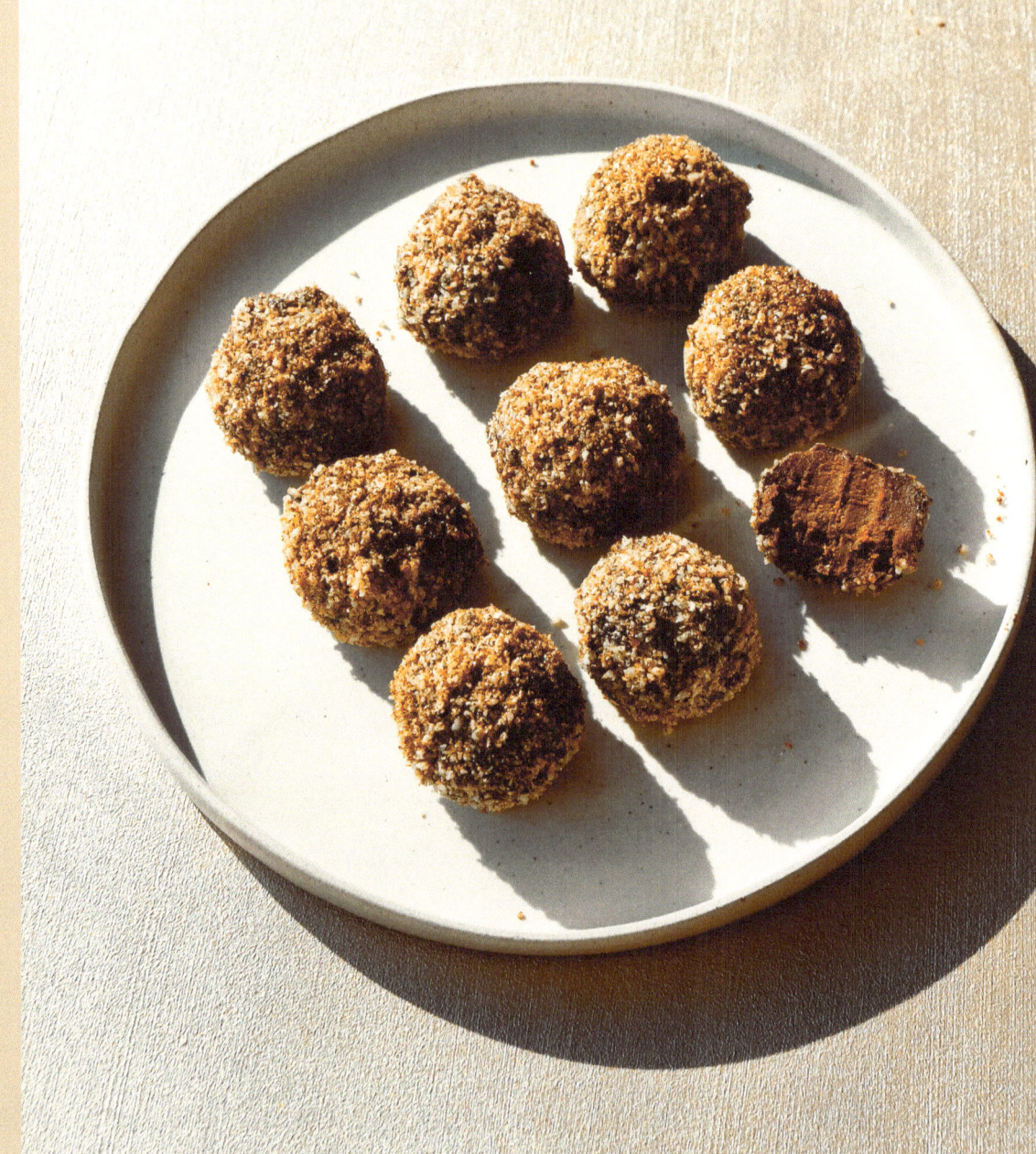

Heliodor known as "gift from sun" in greek. Although these truffles are not Swedish, they have potential to be famous in the near future with its unique flavour.

They contain 70% raw cacao mass gianduja cream, rolled in our solar plexus crumb, infused lavender, bergamot & rosemary.

Designed for the third chakra.

Time - 20 min prep + 10 hrs dehydration
Serves - 12-14 balls

TRUFFLES

165 g almond butter
70 g dark chocolate (70% cacao mass)
15 ml virgin coconut oil
30 ml maple syrup
A pinch pink himalayan salt

SOLAR PLEXUS CRUMB

40 g chopped walnuts
20 g chopped brazil nuts
30 g coconut sugar
5 ml vanilla extract
1/2 tsp cinnamon powder
1/8 tsp clove powder
1/8 tsp nutmeg powder
1/8 tsp pink himalayan salt
2 drops rosemary essential oil
2 drops bergamot essential oil
1 drop lavender essential oil

ENROBING

90 g melted raw chocolate

SOLAR PLEXUS CRUMB

Soak walnuts and brazil nuts together for 2 hours then rinse well and strain.

Place them along with the rest of ingredients in a food processor, fitted with an S blade and process until a chunky texture is achieved. Spread mixture over a dehydrator sheet lined parchment paper. Once dried, transfer mixture in an airtight container, allow to cool for 10 minutes. Then put in the refrigerator. It is ready to roll your truffles. Mixture can be stored in the fridge up to 2 months.

TRUFFLES

Melt the raw chocolate over the bain marie.

Meanwhile place the almond butter, coconut oil, maple and salt in your food processor. Mix together. Once the chocolate is melted, pour over the mixture, blend again.

Using your hands, make 14 equal small balls from the dough. Freeze the balls for 15 minutes after you shaped.

ASSEMBLY

Roll the truffles in melted chocolate and then roll in the solar plexus crumb. Refrigerate at least 40 minutes before serving.

MANGO CHOCOLATE TART

RAW FIKA

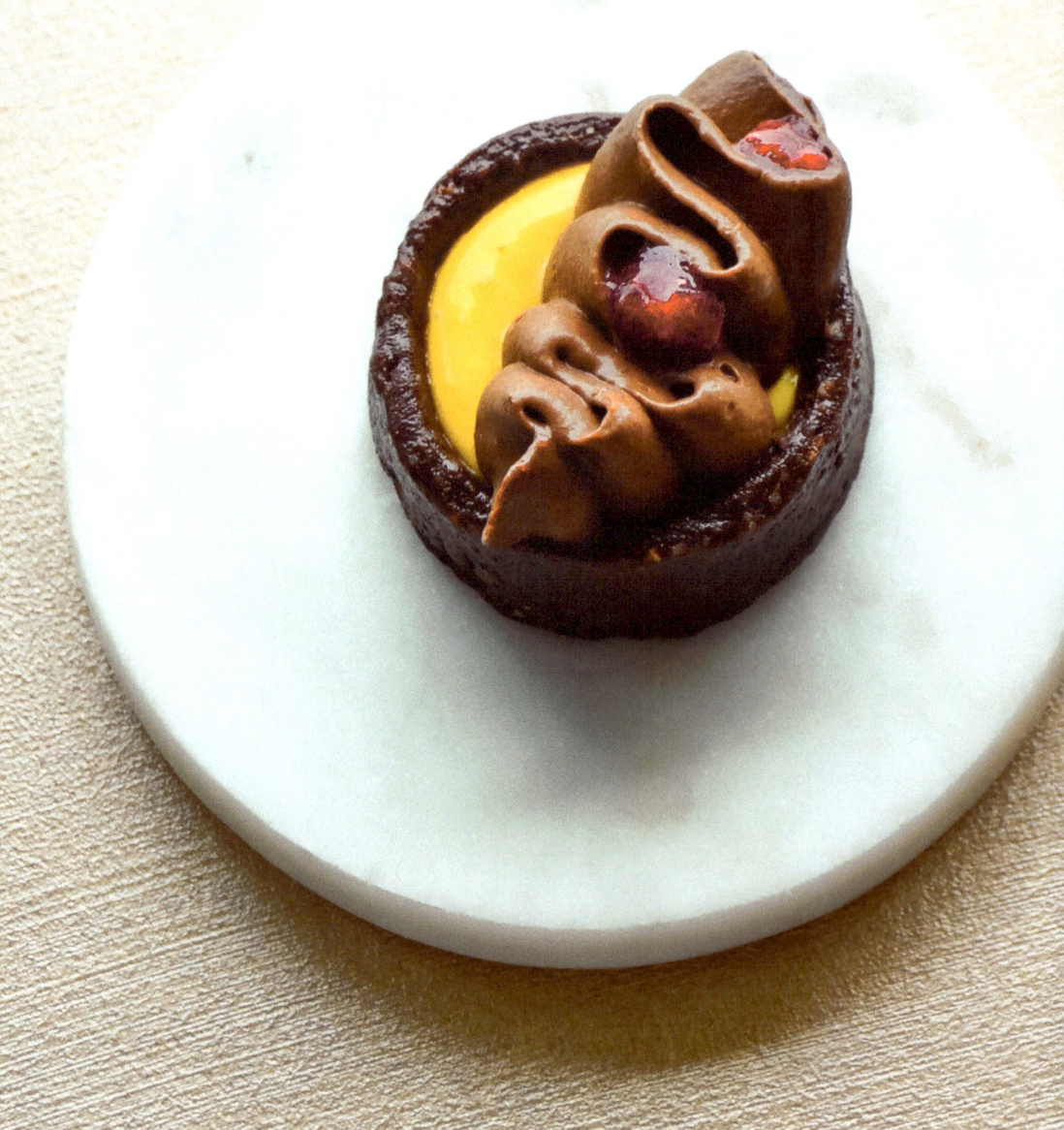

Time - 1 hour + 1 hour setting
Serves - 6

Chocolate Crust
100 g almond flour
50 g coconut sugar powdered
15 g raw cacao powder
50 g raw chocolate melted (min 56% cacao mass)
7 ml tamari or coconut aminos
15 ml water as needed to bind

Mango Cream
100 g ripe mango
50 g ripe banana
90 g coconut cream
45 ml coconut oil melted
30 ml maple syrup
1/4 tsp turmeric powder
A pinch pink himalayan salt

Cherry Jam
100 g raw cherry jam (page 29)

Avocado Chocolate Frosting
1 ripe hass type avocado
90 g coconut cream
30 ml coconut milk
15 g raw cacao powder
60 ml maple syrup
45 ml coconut oil melted
A pinch of pink himalayan salt

CHOCOLATE CRUST
Place almond flour, coconut sugar and raw cacao powder in a food processor, pulse to mix.
Then add the rest of ingredients and blend together. The mix should come together, but not be so moist that it forms into a ball in the machine. Line the cake tins (Round tart tins 4.5 cm wide and 2 cm long) with cling film, or use a silicone baking tin, and press the crust into the base, bringing it up the sides. Dampen your fingers with coconut oil as needed to smooth it out and keep it from sticking to your hands. Repeat the process for the rest. Pop in the freezer while you make the filling or dehydrate the crust in the prepared tart tins lined with a strip of greaseproof. It can be made two ways.

MANGO CREAM
To make mango cream, place all ingredients in a blender except coconut oil. Blend until puree. Then add melted coconut oil, process again until you get silky smooth texture.

AVOCADO CHOCOLATE FROSTING
Place all ingredients in a blender except coconut oil, blend together, lastly add melted coconut oil, blend until silky smooth. Refrigerate for 2 hours before piping process.

ASSEMBLY
Unmold the crust.
Pour mixture in the chocolate crust. Freeze while making cherry jam and avocado frosting.
Make the cherry jam (page 39) according the instructions given on the pages. Place the avocado frosting in a piping bag with Wilton 125 tip, decorate the tart with the frosting.
Using another pipping bag without tip, drop some small cherry jam dots between avocado chocolate frosting.

BLUEBERRY CHOCOLATE BROWNIE BITES

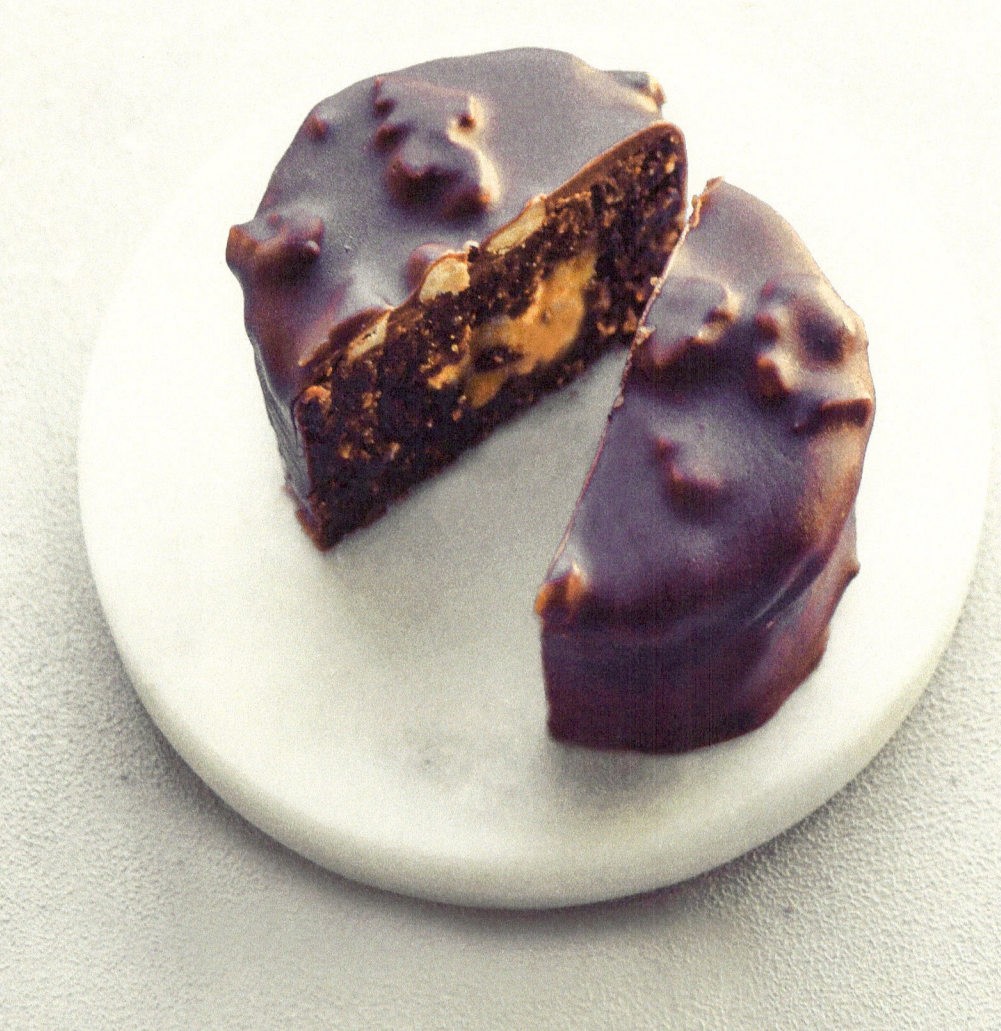

Time - 20 min prep + 1 hour setting
Serves - 15 pieces

Brownie
95 g dehydrated cookie base (page 28)
55 g raw blueberry jam (page 29)
75 g dried raisins soaked
30 ml virgin coconut oil melted
10 g raw cacao powder
A pinch pink himalayan salt

Filling
20 g hazelnut butter

Enrobing
100 g raw chocolate melted
15 ml virgin coconut oil melted
20 g walnuts chopped

BROWNIE
Place the cookie base in a food processor, run into flour. Then add the blueberry jam, soaked rinsed raisins, cacao powder, salt and melted coconut oil, blend together until the dough comes together.

ASSEMBLY
Divide mixture into 4 pieces (just leave 2 teaspoon dough from each piece to cover the hazelnut butter hole later) , transfer to 5 cm cake tins lined parchment paper. Press down with your fingers and then with the back of a teaspoon. Using your finger carve a hole in the middle, put a teaspoon hazelnut butter in the hole. Cover the top with brownie. Flatten the top out as much as possible. Repeat the process for the rest of pieces. Freeze for 2 hours.

Meanwhile melt the raw chocolate and coconut oil using bain marie. Once melted, add chopped walnuts and stir well to combine together.

Remove the brownies from the freezer, place the brownie on the back of a 3 cm small bowl or cooling tray. Pour the the chocolate over the brownie, make sure all parts of the brownie covered well with the chocolate. Repeat the process for the rest. Refrigerate for 45-40 minutes before serving.

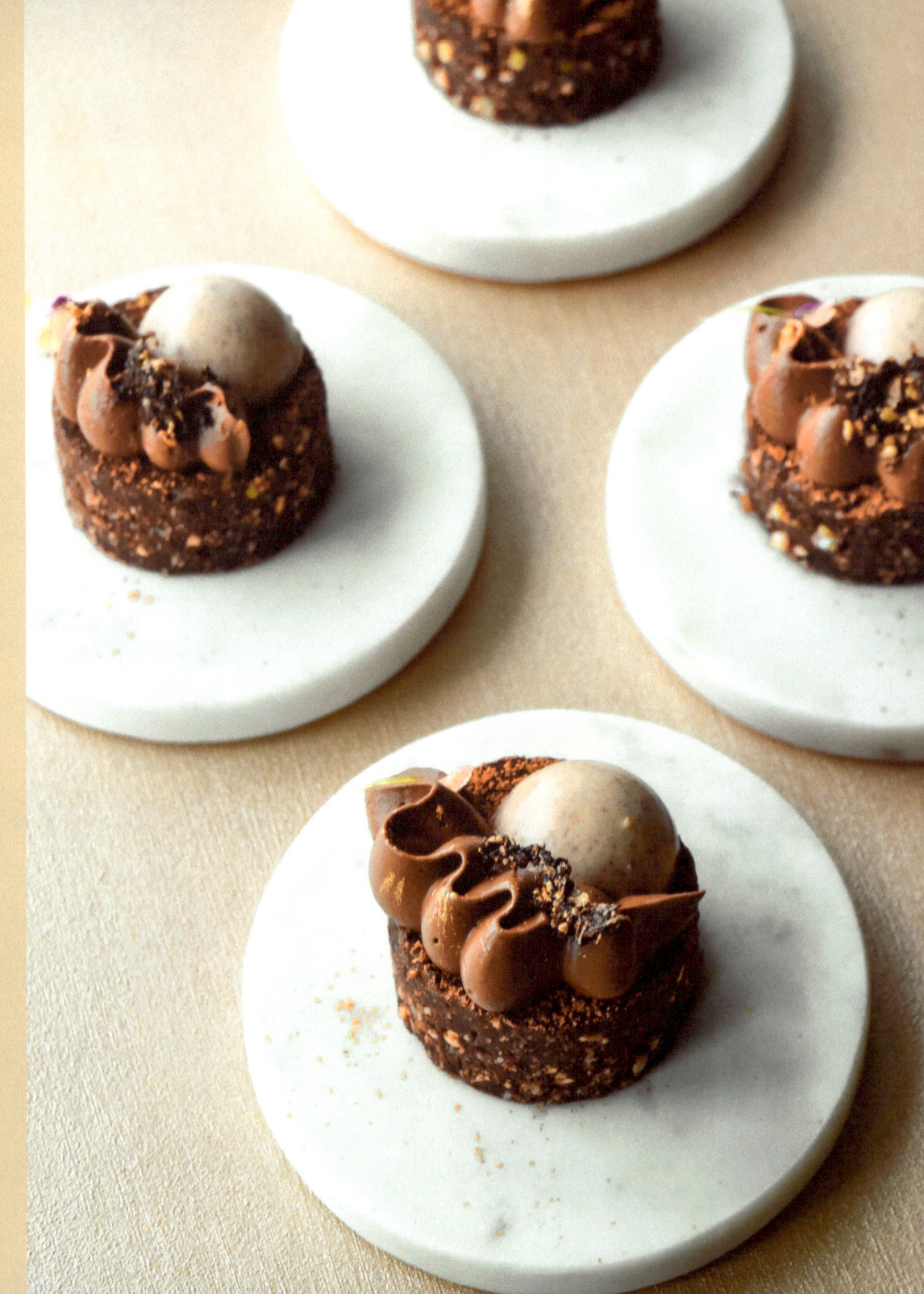

RAW FIKA

BROWNIE

HAZELNUT CREAM, AVOCADO FROSTING & WAKAME CRISP

Time - 1 hour + 4 hours dehydration + 3 hours setting

Serves - 6-8 person

Brownie Base

120 g sprouted rolled oats
60 g raw cacao powder
60 g raw almond butter
25 g buckini
50 ml virgin coconut oil melted
100 g dried raisins soaked
70 ml maple syrup
10 ml coconut aminos or tamari

Hazelnut Cream

100 g raw hazelnuts soaked
60 g coconut cream
15 ml virgin coconut oil melted
2 drops medicine flower hazelnut extract
A pinch of pink himalayan salt

Avocado Frosting

1 ripe hass type avocado
90 g coconut cream
30 ml coconut milk
15 g raw cacao powder
60 ml maple syrup
45 ml virgin coconut oil melted
A pinch of pink himalayan salt

Mushroom Wakame Crisp

200 g chesnut mushrooms
10 g sesame seeds
15 ml extra virgin olive oil
7 g atlantic atlantic wakame flakes
15 g coconut sugar powdered
15 ml coconut aminos

BROWNIE BASE

Place the rolled oat flour and raw cacao powder in a food processor. Mix together until well combined. Then add the maple, dried soaked raisins, coconut aminos, melted coconut oil. Process until the dough comes together. When you press with your fingers it should be come together easily.
Once done, add buckini and knead with your hands. Divide the dough between a 8 cm round cake tins lined parchment paper. Put 4-5 tbsp of dough for each mold and press and smooth. Depending on the amount of dough you put, you will get 6-8 cakes. Freeze for about 30-40 minutes.

HAZELNUT CREAM

Place soaked drained hazelnuts in the blender. Add rest of the ingredients except coconut oil. Process to get a silky smooth mixture. Lastly add coconut oil and blend again to combine. Pour mixture into 3 cm round silicon molds. Freeze for 2-3 hours or until completely firm.

AVOCADO FROSTING

Make the avocado frosting acccording to the instructions given on the page 30. Taste it, adjust the salt or maple as needed.

MUSHROOM WAKAME CRISP

Brush and clean your mushrooms and place in the food processor. Add the olive oil, coconut aminos and coconut sugar. Run until you get slightly rice-like texture. Remove the mixture from the food processor into a small bowl, add the sesame seeds and wakame flakes. Stir well.
Place on a lined dehydrator tray and dehydrate at 42°C for 2 hours then flip onto mesh tray, continue to dehydrate another 2 hours or until completely dry. Remove from dehydrator, let them cool for 15 minutes. Then they're ready to use in your recipes. Can be stored in airtight container or mason jars up to 2-3 months.

ASSEMBLY

Once hazelnut cream bubbles are chilled, place the rounds on the brownies. Transfer the avocado cream in a piping bag with Wilton 125 tip, decorate the brownie with the frosting.
Using a chef tweezer, leave some crisps over the avocado frosting. Decorate with edible gold and flowers if desired.

ALLA HJÄRTANS DAG TÅRTA

RASPBERRY VALENTINES DAY CAKE

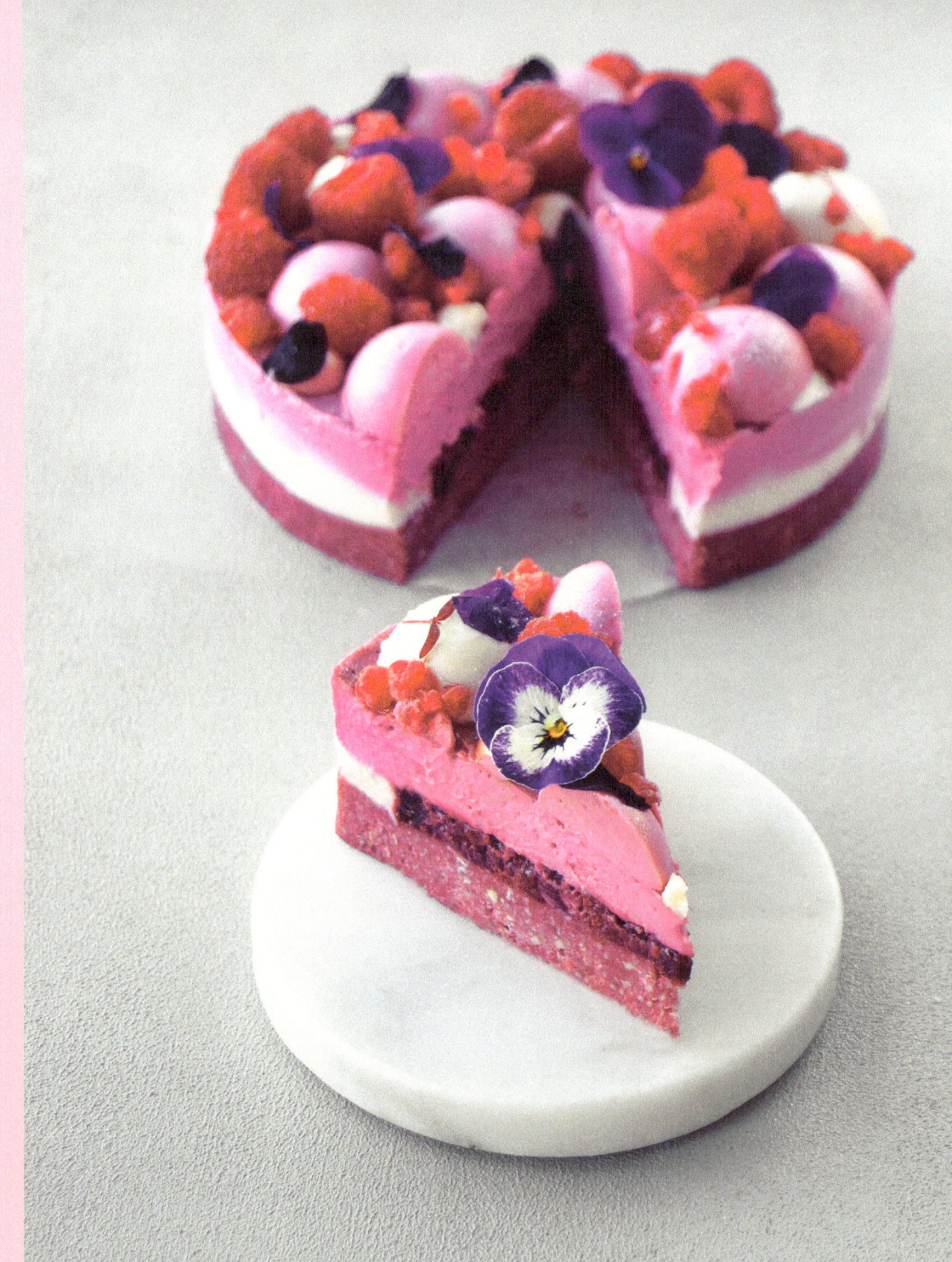

Time - 2 hours prep + 6 hours dehydration + 6-8 hours setting
Serves - 6 slices

Crust
60 g tigernut flour
30 g sprouted oat flour
20 g desiccated coconut
20 g dried mulberries
20 ml virgin coconut oil melted
30 g tahini
10 g beetroot powder
10 g raspberry powder
5 ml vanilla extract
7 ml lemon juice
1/4 tsp ground cardamom
1/8 tsp pink himalayan salt

Coconut Pastry Cream
85 g young coconut meat
75 g coconut cream
50 ml coconut nectar syrup
23 g freeze dried raspberry powder
50 g fresh raspberries
35 ml virgin coconut oil melted
15 g cacao butter melted
15 ml lemon juice
5 ml vanilla extract
5 g sunflower lecithin powder
1/8 tsp pink himalayan salt

Raspberry Jam
150 g defrosted raspberries
10 g chia seeds
10 ml lemon juice
20 ml coconut nectar syrup

Frosting Bubbles
70 g young coconut meat
60 ml coconut cream
40 ml coconut nectar syrup
20 ml virgin coconut oil melted
20 g raw cacao butter melted
15 ml lemon juice
5 ml vanilla extract
5 g sunflower lecithin powder
1/8 tsp pink himalayan salt

Decoration
Fresh raspberries
Purple pansies
Edible pink gold powder

RASPBERRY JAM

First start by making raspberry jam. You need to start making it overnight or 6 hours beforehand.
Defrost raspberries in a bowl, add chia seeds, lemon juice and coconut nectar. Smash with a fork. Place in the dehydrator, and dehydrate at 42°C for about 6 hours or it becomes a thick jam-like consistency. Then set aside.

CRUST

Place tigernut flour, sprouted oat flour, desiccated coconut, dried mulberries, salt, beet powder, raspberry powder and cardamom in a food processor. Mix to combine together. Then add tahini, melted coconut oil, lemon juice and vanilla extract. Process until dough comes together. Transfer dough in a 15 cm round cake mould line parchment paper. Press down with your fingers, then flatten out with a back of spoon as much as possible. A good molding makes the cake flawless. So do not rush the leveling process at this stage. Place the crust in the fridge while you are making the filling cream.

COCONUT PASTRY CREAM

To make filling, place coconut meat, coconut cream, coconut nectar, lemon juice, vanilla extract, lecithin powder and salt in a high speed blender. Blend until smooth.

ASSEMBLY

Remove cake crust from the refrigerator. Place a 10 cm round cake tin (without a bottom) on the middle of crust. Pour 1/4 of the coconut pastry cream into the 5 cm area outside the 10 cm in the middle.
Tap the mold gently so that it is evenly distributed.
Now put the jam into the middle of the 10 cm mold. Flatten with the back of a spoon. Place the mold in the freezer.
Remove it after 20 minutes. Now gently pull out the 10 cm round mold that you placed in the middle.
The cream is almost solidified but tends to flow slightly to fill the gap in between. If it is completely solidified, you can add a few teaspoon of cream to combine it with the border of the jam layer. Freeze for 1-2 hours until it is thick enough to pour another layer so layers will not blend together.

Place back to the blender, you have poured 1/4 of the mixture to the crust. Add raspberry powder and beet powder to the rest of the mixture. Blend until smooth.

Once time is up, remove the cake from the freezer. Pour the rest of the mixture over the coconut pastry cream and jam layer. Tap to to the mould slightly to prevent bubbles. Freeze again at least 5 hours before unmoulding.

Meanwhile, start making bubbles. Place coconut meat, coconut cream, coconut nectar, lemon juice, vanilla extract, salt and sunflower lecithin. Blend together until well combined and smooth.
For the bubbles I use a special mold called "Pralinform halvklot" from Pufz Sweden, it is 35 pieces with a diameter of 3 cm and 24 pieces with a diameter of 1.5 cm.
This mold is very versatile, not only for bubble decoration, but also for the middle layers of cakes and layered bliss balls. I used it in the middle of the Japanese matcha hemispherical cakes in this book. Also used it in the ferrawro recipe in my "Mad About Raw" book.

You don't need to fill all the pieces if you are making a 15 cm medium cake. But if you are planning to make a bigger one, it would be better to use all the bubbles in the mold.
If you don't have small eclipse molds, they can easily be replaced by other silicone molds in 3 cm and 1.5 cm sizes at your hand. If you don't have any, check on Amazon to see available options. You can also pipe the cream with your favorite nozzle instead decorating with bubbles. Feel free to use which one is best for you.

Pour the white cream in the bubbles. Fill 6-8 bubbles depending on your choice. Then back to blender, add beet powder and raspberry powder, blend until well mixed. Divide the pink cream between bubbles. Freeze the mold at least 4 hours until the bubbles are thick enough.

Once time is up, remove the cake and bubbles from the freezer. Unmould the cake and bubbles. Place the bubbles on top of cake as shown in the picture. Fill the gaps with fresh raspberries and edible purple and blue pansies.
Slice with a sharp and warm chef knife and serve!

TIP: If you take enough time to chill your cake before cutting, you can make slicing even easier by running your knife under hot water before using. It's important that you heat and properly clean the blade of your knife in between each cut. So, before you begin cutting, briefly soak the blade in a container of warm water or running your knife under hot water before using. Then, wipe dry the blade with a paper towel. The warm blade will help with cutting into your cake.

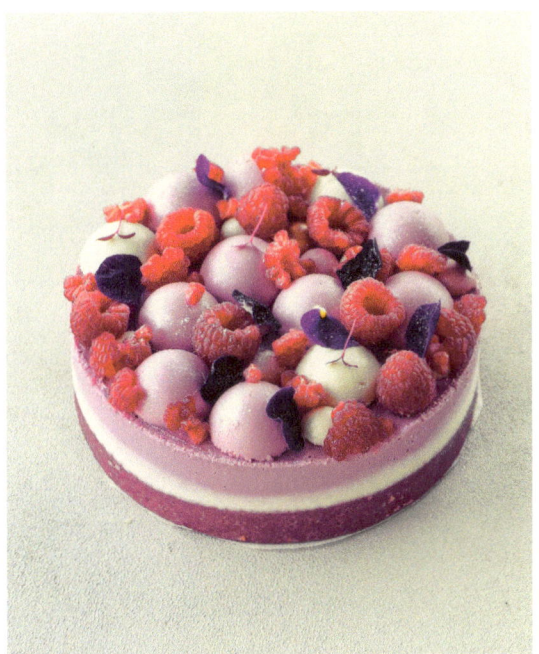

PANDAN AVOCADO PISTACHIO COCONUT FRAMBOISE SQUARES

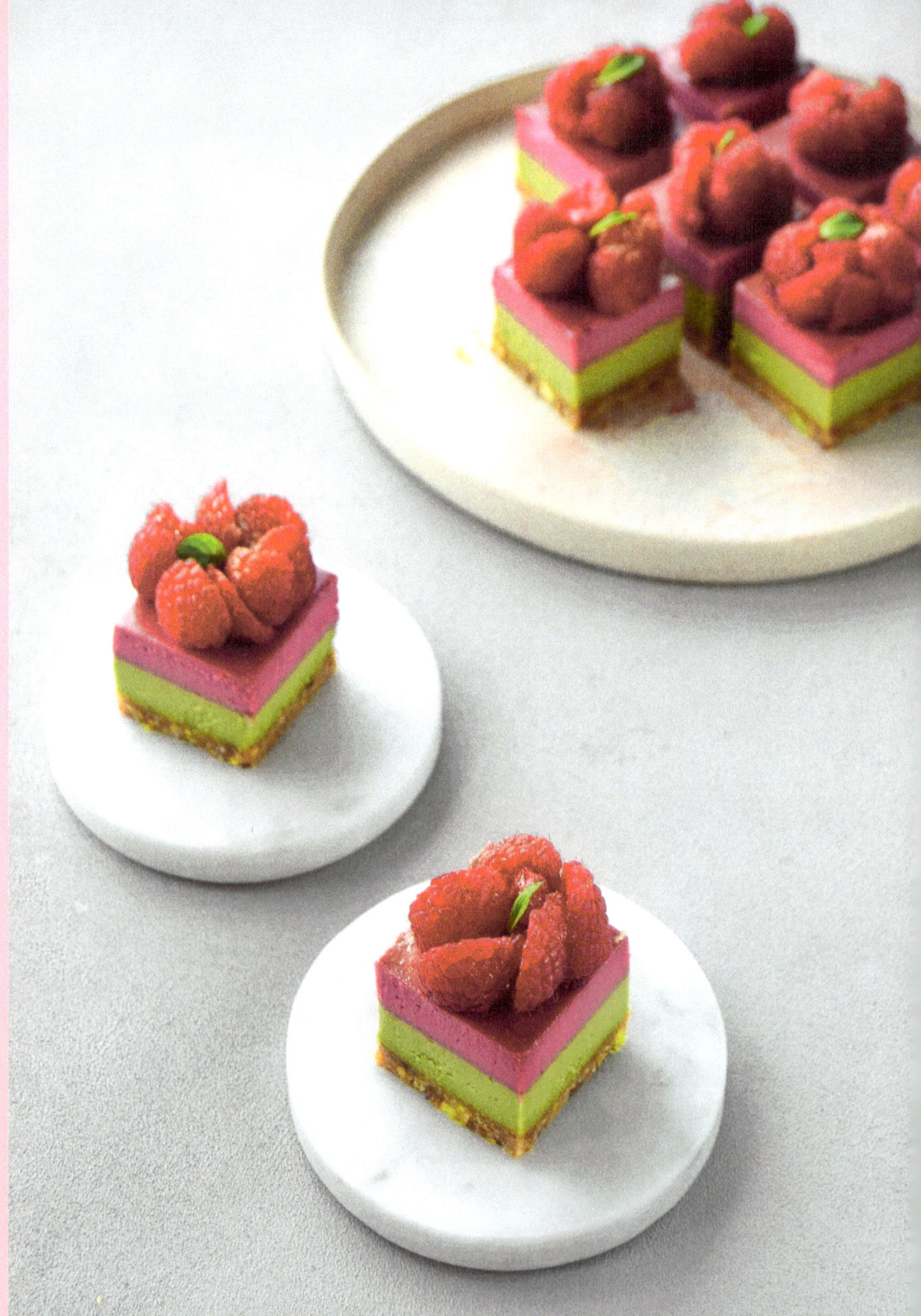

The fact is, raw pandan tastes quite grassy. But when it's prepared with various desserts, it has a very unique taste that can be described as a creamy coconut, banana-leafy, slightly nutty flavor. In this combination, I blended pandan with coconut, pistachio and avocado which is my most loved signature flavours. It is light, creamy and tastes heavenly. Layered with bright framboise cream. The floral, sweet flavor of the pandan goes amazing with the fresh, tangy flavor of the raspberry.

Time - 1 hour prep + 5 hours setting
Serves - 9 Squares

Crust
45 g coconut sugar powdered
82 g almond flour
10 g coconut flour
25 g pistachios
5 g flaxseeds
15 ml virgin coconut oil melted
10 ml coconut milk
A pinch pink himalayan salt

Pistachio Pandan Filling
55 g pistachio soaked
55 g young coconut meat
50 g avocado meat
40 ml coconut milk
55 ml maple syrup
50 ml virgin coconut oil melted
15 ml lemon juice
15 g pandan powder
A pinch pink himalayan salt

Raspberry Cheesecake Filling
75 g cashews soaked
70 g coconut cream
30 ml maple syrup
40 ml virgin coconut oil melted
10 ml lemon juice
15 g freeze dried raspberry powder
5 g beetroot powder
5 ml vanilla extract
A pinch pink himalayan salt

Decoration
140 g fresh raspberries
Small fresh mint leaves
Edible gold powder to dust

CRUST

To make crust, first prepare the pistachios. To remove pistachio skins, first remove the nuts from the shells. Cover the nuts with water and let them stand for 30 minutes. Drain the water and place the nuts in a dish towel. Rub them vigorously - the skins will slip right off. Then dehydrate the pistachios at 46°C for 6-8 hours or completely dried.

The next, place coconut sugar, almond flour, coconut flour and salt in your food processor, mix together.

Then add melted coconut oil and coconut milk, blend together until dough slightly comes together. Lastly add dehydrated whole pistachios and flaxseeds, pulse twice (we want some crunchy big pieces inside the dough) and remove dough from the food processor. Knead with your hands. Transfer to a 15x15 cm square cake tin lined parchment paper. Press down with your hands and with a back of spoon to flatten out. Keep in the fridge while making the fillings.

PISTACHIO PANDAN

To make pistachio pandan filling, remove the pistachios from the shells, soak for 15 minutes. Then rinse and transfer into the blender.

Cut the avocado in half. Grasp the outer dark layer or skin and pull it away from the inner green flesh of the fruit. If some of the darker almost black portions of the skin remain on the green flesh of the fruit, simply cut them away.

Add young coconut meat, avocado meat, coconut milk, maple, lemon juice, salt and pandan powder into the blender. Blend together until smooth. Lastly add melted coconut oil, process again until well combined.

Pour the pistachio pandan mixture over the crust. Gently tap the mold in order to prevent bubbles. Freeze for 1-2 hours or so until it is thick enough to pour another layer.

RASPBERRY FILLING

Meanwhile, start making raspberry cheesecake filling. Place soaked rinsed cashews in a blender. Add the rest of ingredients except coconut oil. Blend together until silky smooth.

If the mixture is too thick, add the water you soaked the cashew nuts in, 1 tbsp (15 ml) at a time. Lastly add melted coconut oil, blend well.

ASSEMBLY

Once time is up, remove the cake from the freezer, pour the raspberry filling over the pistachio filling. Freeze for 4-5 hours before cutting.
Cut your cake into 9 equal squares.

Dust some raspberry powder on top to make an "mirror" color effect, and decorate with fresh raspberries and mint if desired.

It keeps well in the fridge for 3 to 4 days. You can also freeze it for up to a month. (It's usually gone by the end of the day, though...)

KÅLRABBIGRÖT - KOHLRABI PORRIDGE

Time - 30 min prep
Serves - 2

Gröt means porridge, a warming food made from oats or rice and water or milk and beloved in Sweden since Viking times. Our raw version made of kohlrabi, it is flavourful, vibrant and nourishing. Other great alternatives can be rutabaga and cauliflower.

Ingredients

135 g kohlrabi
50 g almond butter
80 ml fresh orange juice
7 ml coconut oil
15 ml maple syrup
1/8 tsp ground cardamom
4 g cinnamon powder
1/2 tsp vanilla bean powder
1/4 tsp ground ginger or grated fresh ginger
A pinch of licorice salt
Orange zest, almond butter to serve

INSTRUCTIONS

Peel your kohlrabi and cut it into chunks around 1"wide. Blend chunks in a food processor until they break down to look rice-like. Transfer them to a nut milk bag in a bowl and squeeze out any excess liquid. Discard the liquid and put the rice in a clean bowl. Blend up almond butter, orange juice, maple, cinnamon, cardamom, vanilla, ginger and a pinch of salt in a high-speed blender until smooth. Add to the kohrabi rice. Combine well. Transfer mixture in a large bowl. If you have dehydrator and want to eat it warm: Cover the bowl with a cling film, dehydrate at 42-46°C in the dehydrator for 30-40 minutes or until warm. Pour 1 tsp coconut oil in the middle of the bowl and let it melt for 2-3 minutes. Peel the orange, put orange zest on your bowl, along with the raisins. Dust some cinnamon powder if desired. Enjoy.

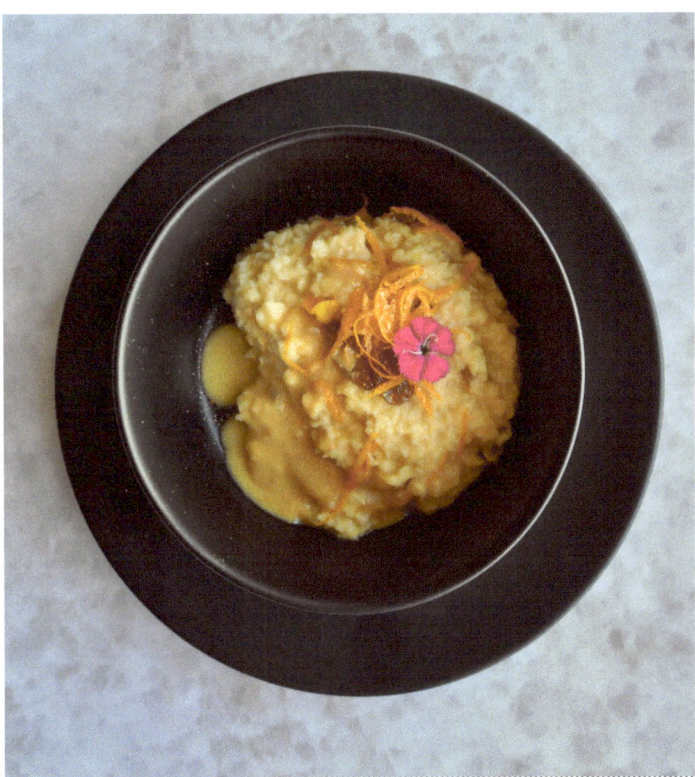

KOKOSFLARN
COCONUT CRISP COOKIES

A chewy oatmeal cookies called "havreflarn", made mainly with oats, are one of "Sju sorters kakor" (seven kind of cookies) very popular in Sweden. In recent years, versions made with coconut have also become quite common.
These Swedish coconut cookies "kokosflarn" that come as singles or in pairs, sandwiched together by a layer of dark chocolate. If you want to make oat version, just replace desiccated coconut with oatmeal.

Time - 1 hour + 12 hrs dehydration
Serves - 10 cookies

Ingredients
60 g desiccated coconut
60 g almond flour
15 g coconut flour
50 ml maple syrup
15 ml virgin coconut oil melted
15 g raw cacao butter melted
1 tsp vanilla extract

INSTRUCTIONS
In a large bowl, combine all ingredients and stir well. Refrigerate the bowl for 30 minutes. This will help you to form the cookies.

Once cooled, using a tablespoon or icecream spoon, spoon rounds of the dough, transfer to a 5-cm round food molding (we use from Ateco brand) with a fitted press. Press down with the fitted press.
Transfer to a dehydrator sheet. Dehydrate for 10-12 hours or overnight until completely dried.

You can also eat them without dehydrating. They are delicious either way. but dehydrating is more ideal for long-term storage and for a crunch in real cookie texture.

(See the picture on right page)

GRÄDDBULLE
SWEDISH FLUFFY CREAM BUNS

Time - 1 hrs + 2 hrs setting
Serves - 10 pieces

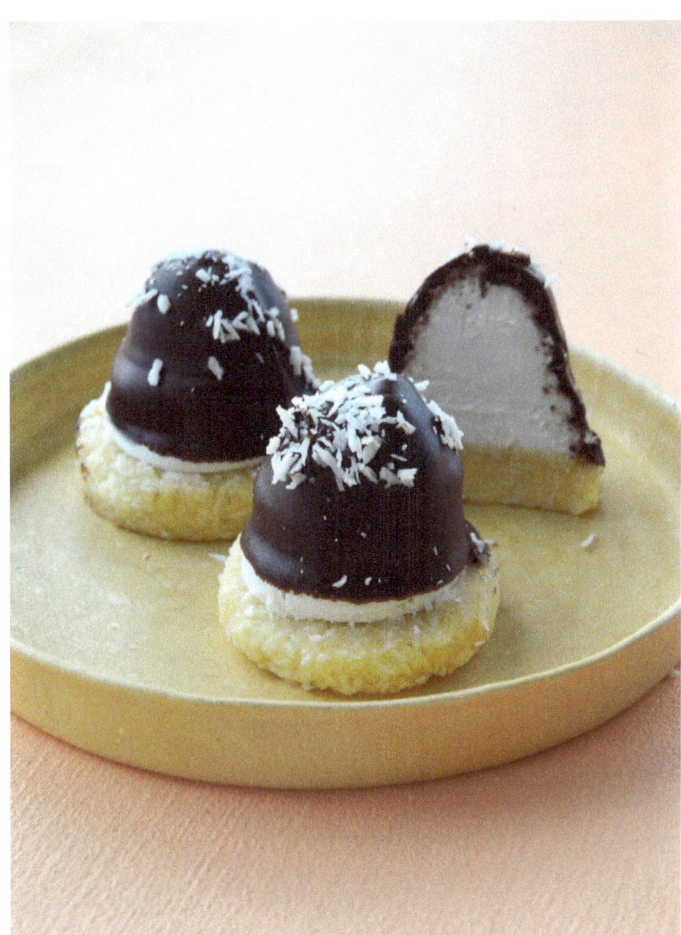

Cream bun, coconut bun or foam ball - this nostalgic Swedish treat has many names. Making your own cream buns is well worth it because they turn out heavenly good with all natural ingredients and just as fluffy as you want them.

INGREDIENTS

1 batch kokosflarn (see on the left page)
400 ml coconut cream
50 ml virgin coconut oil melted
60 ml irish moss gel
50 ml coconut nectar syrup
15 ml lemon juice
2 tsp vanilla extract
A pinch pink himalayan salt
200 g raw chocolate melted for dipping + 15 ml coconut oil
Desiccated coconut for garnish

INSTRUCTIONS

Make kokosflarn according to recipe on the left page. To make cream, place coconut cream, irish moss gel, lemon juice, melted coconut oil, coconut nectar, vanilla extract, and salt in a deep bowl. Whisk for couple of minutes until whipped well. Transfer to a piping bag with Wilton 12 round tip. Squeeze the filling to make a fluffy peak on the each kokosflarn. Put them in the freezer.

Melt the chocolate, add the coconut oil and mix together. Then dip the cream balls in the chocolate. Sprinkle desiccated coconut.

ORANGE COFFEE FLAVOURED CAKE BARS

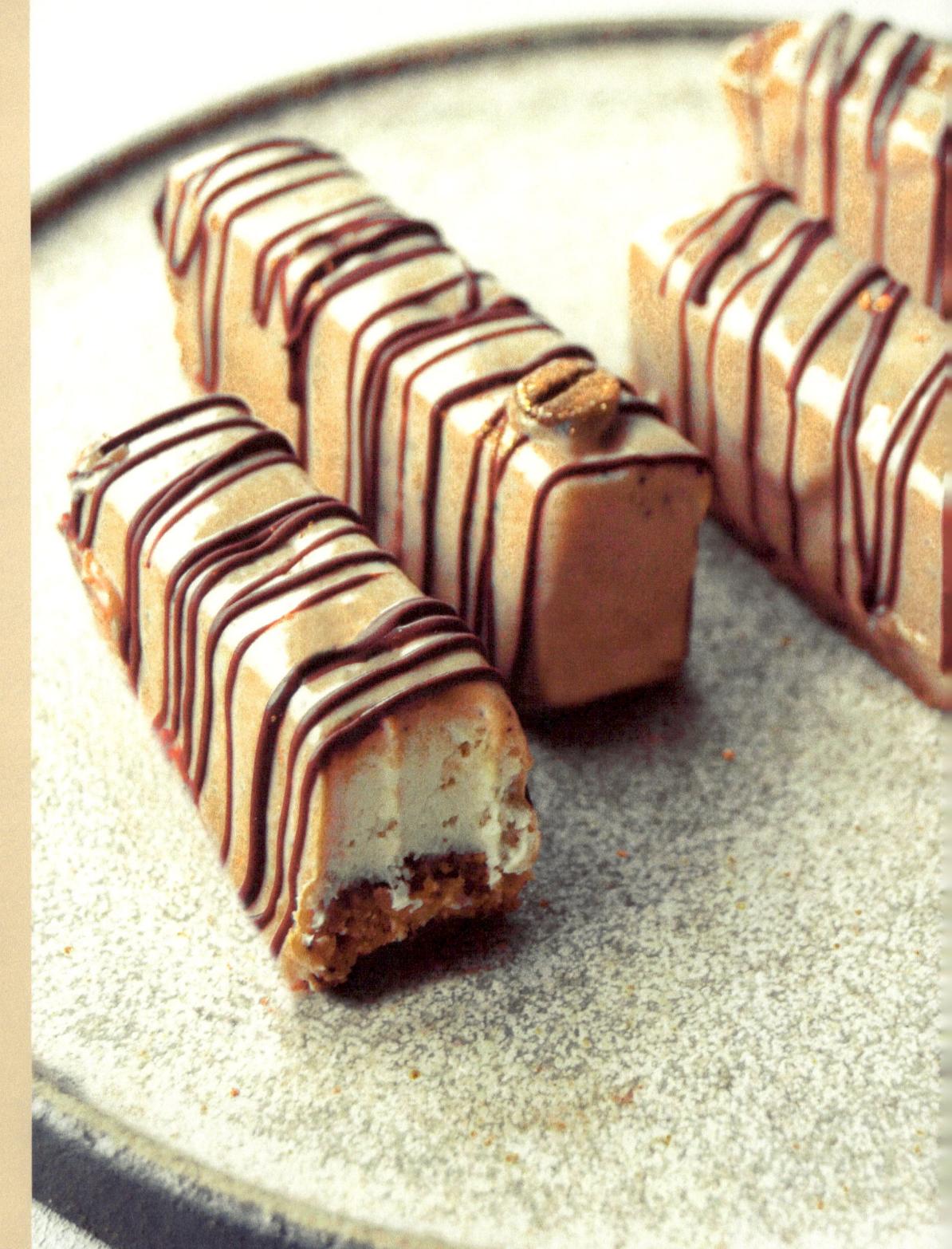

Orange Coffee Glaze

- 90 g cashews soaked
- 65 ml freshly brewed warm coffee
- 30 g coconut sugar powdered
- 40 ml virgin coconut oil melted
- 15 ml maple syrup
- 7 ml lemon juice
- 5 g ground coffee beans
- 1/8 tsp pink himalayan salt
- 6-7 drops orange essential oil

Crust

- 40 g hazelnut flour
- 65 g hazelnut butter
- 40 g oat flour
- 40 g dehydrated activated buckwheats
- 15 ml maple syrup
- 30 ml water
- 30 ml melted coconut oil
- 2 g cinnamon powder
- 1/8 tsp pink himalayan salt
- 4-5 drops orange essential oil

Cream Filling

- 90 g cashews soaked
- 95 g coconut cream
- 15 ml coconut milk
- 50 ml maple syrup
- 45 ml virgin coconut oil melted
- 7 ml lemon juice
- A pinch pink himalayan salt

Chocolate Ganache

- 35 g raw chocolate melted (53% cacao mass)
- 30 g coconut cream
- 10 g virgin coconut oil melted

Time - 50 min prep + 4 hours setting

Serves - 9-10 bars

CRUST

Add hazelnut flour, oat flour, buckwheats, cinnamon powder and salt into a food processor. Mix together. Then add coconut oil, hazelnut butter, orange essential oil, maple and water. Process until dough comes together. Transfer to a 15 cm square cake mold. Press with the back of a spoon, flatten as much as possible. Let it sit in the fridge while making the cream filling.

CREAM FILLING

Add cashews, coconut cream, coconut milk, lemon juice, salt and maple into your blender. Blend until you get a smooth mixture. Then add melted coconut oil. Blend again until incomparated. Pour over the crust, freeze for 4 hours.

ORANGE COFFEE GLAZE

Add cashews, freshly brewed warm coffee, coconut sugar, maple, lemon juice, salt, essential oil and ground coffee beans. Blend until you get a smooth mixture. Then add melted coconut oil, blend until incomparated well. Transfer the glaze into a container with a diameter just slightly wider than the 15 cm cake bars. Let the glaze to set to 31°C.

CHOCOLATE GANACHE

Melt the chocolate over bain marie, mix with coconut cream and coconut oil until incomparated well. Let it cool for 15-20 minutes.

ASSEMBLY

Unmould the frozen cake, cut into 3 inch bars and insert the tip of a small kitchen knife on top of the cake bars. Gently dip each bar into orange coffee glaze, make sure the sides are well coated with the glaze.

Gently scrape the bottom of the bars on a sheet of parchment paper or silicone mat to remove any excess glaze then place it on top of the crust. Place in the fridge for approximatively 3-4 hours. Once cakes are cooled, transfer chocolate ganache in a paper piping cone or a small disposable piping bag and cut a very small tip off the end. Pipe stripes of chocolate on top of each bar. Garnish with some coffee beans or edible gold powder to finish.

JAPANESE MATCHA YUZU CAKES

RAW FIKA

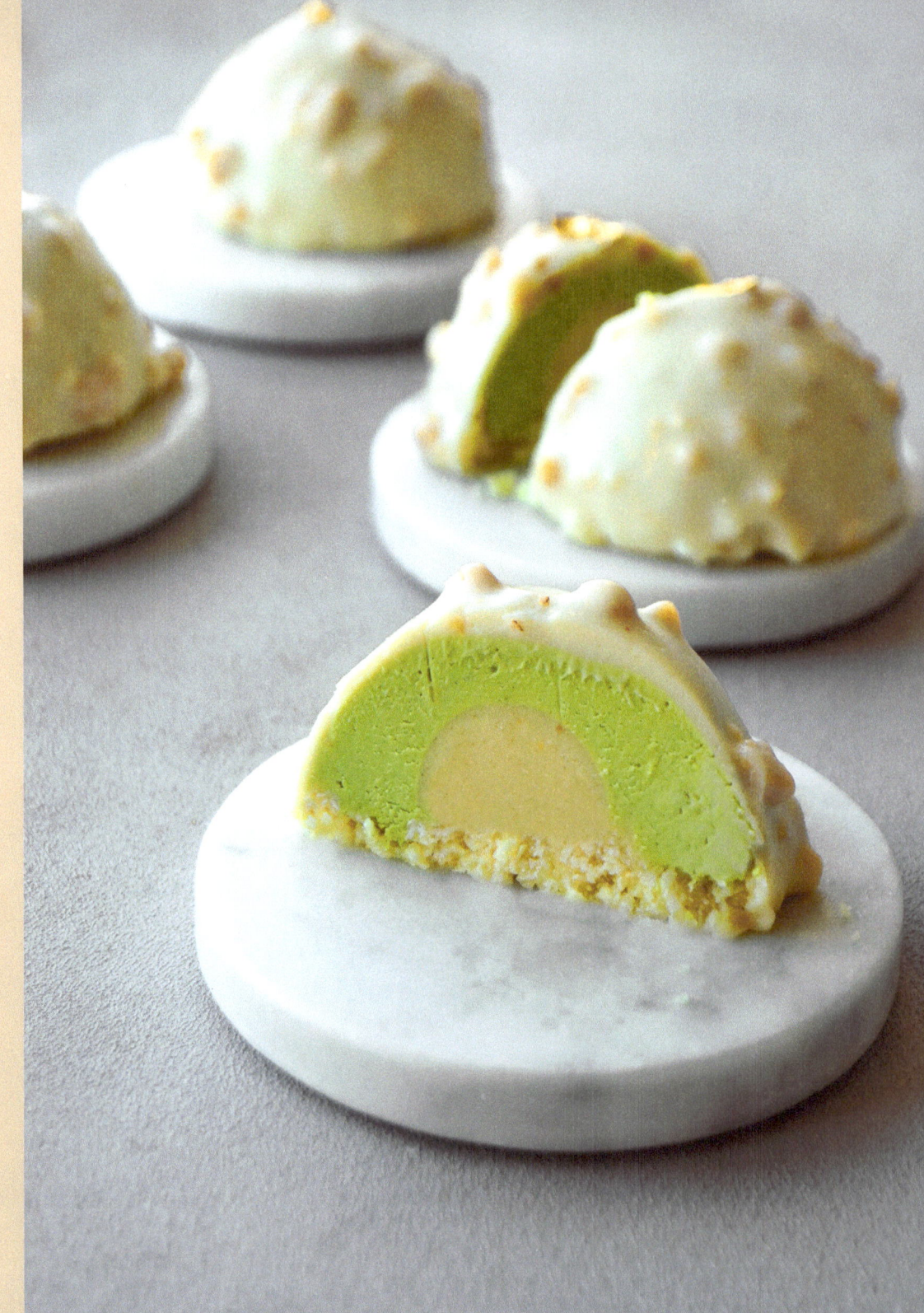

Time - 2 hours prep + 4 hours setting
Serves - 7

Crust
80 g desiccated coconut
30 ml coconut nectar syrup
35 g blanced almond butter
25 g cacao butter melted
1/8 tsp pink himalayan salt

Matcha Yuzu Cream
125 g young coconut meat
50 g coconut cream
30 g yuzu juice
60 ml coconut nectar syrup
4-5 drops yuzu essential oil
1.5 tsp japanese matcha powder
30 ml virgin coconut oil melted
30 g cacao butter melted
1/8 tsp pink himalayan salt

Macadamia Praline
50 g macadamia butter
35 ml coconut nectar syrup
15 g cacao butter melted
15 g coconut cream
A pinch pink himalayan salt

White Chocolate Ganache
100 g cashews soaked
40 ml coconut milk
40 g coconut cream
50 ml coconut nectar syrup
30 ml virgin coconut oil melted
30 g cacao butter melted
7 ml yuzu juice
A pinch pink himalayan salt
30 g chopped macadamia

MACADAMIA PRALINE
Start by making macadamia praline, place all ingredients in a small blender. Blend until smooth. Pour in 3 cm half sphere moulds. Freeze while making matcha yuzu cream.

MATCHA YUZU CREAM
To make matcha yuzu cream, place young coconut meat, coconut cream, yuzu juice, coconut nectar syrup, essential oil and salt into blender. Blend on high speed until smooth. Then add melted cacao butter and coconut oil. Blend again until incorporated well. Divide the mixture into 7 cm half sphere moulds. You will have 7 pieces 7 cm cakes. Do not fill the mould. There should be some space on the top for placing the crust later. Set in the freezer for 10 minutes.

CRUST
Place all crust ingredients in a food processor, blend together. Freeze for 15 minutes then roll between two parchment paper. Using a 7 cm ring cutter, cut the crust. Set aside.

WHITE CHOCOLATE GANACHE
To make white chocolate ganache, place cashews, coconut milk, coconut cream, coconut nectar, yuzu juice and salt. Blend until smooth. Lastly add melted coconut oil and coconut butter, blend again until well incorporated. Let the mixture sit in the fridge for 8-10 minutes. Then whisk well. Add the chopped macadamia in the mixture. Stir well.

ASSEMBLY
Remove macadamia pralines and matcha yuzu moulds from the freezer. Unmould the pralines. Place them in the middle of the matcha yuzu spheres. Gently press with your finger. The end of praline should be at the same line with matcha yuzu cream. Freeze for 2 hours or until completely cooled. Then place the crust layer on the yuzu cream. Freeze for another hour. Remove the domes from the freezer, transfer to a cake rack. Pour the white chocolate ganach over the cakes. Make sure all parts of the cake covered with ganache. Immediately place the rack in the freezer for 20 minutes. Keep in the fridge for 2-3 hours before serving in order to allow developing the flavours.

RAW FIKA

JORDGUBBSTÅRTA

MIDSOMMAR CAKE

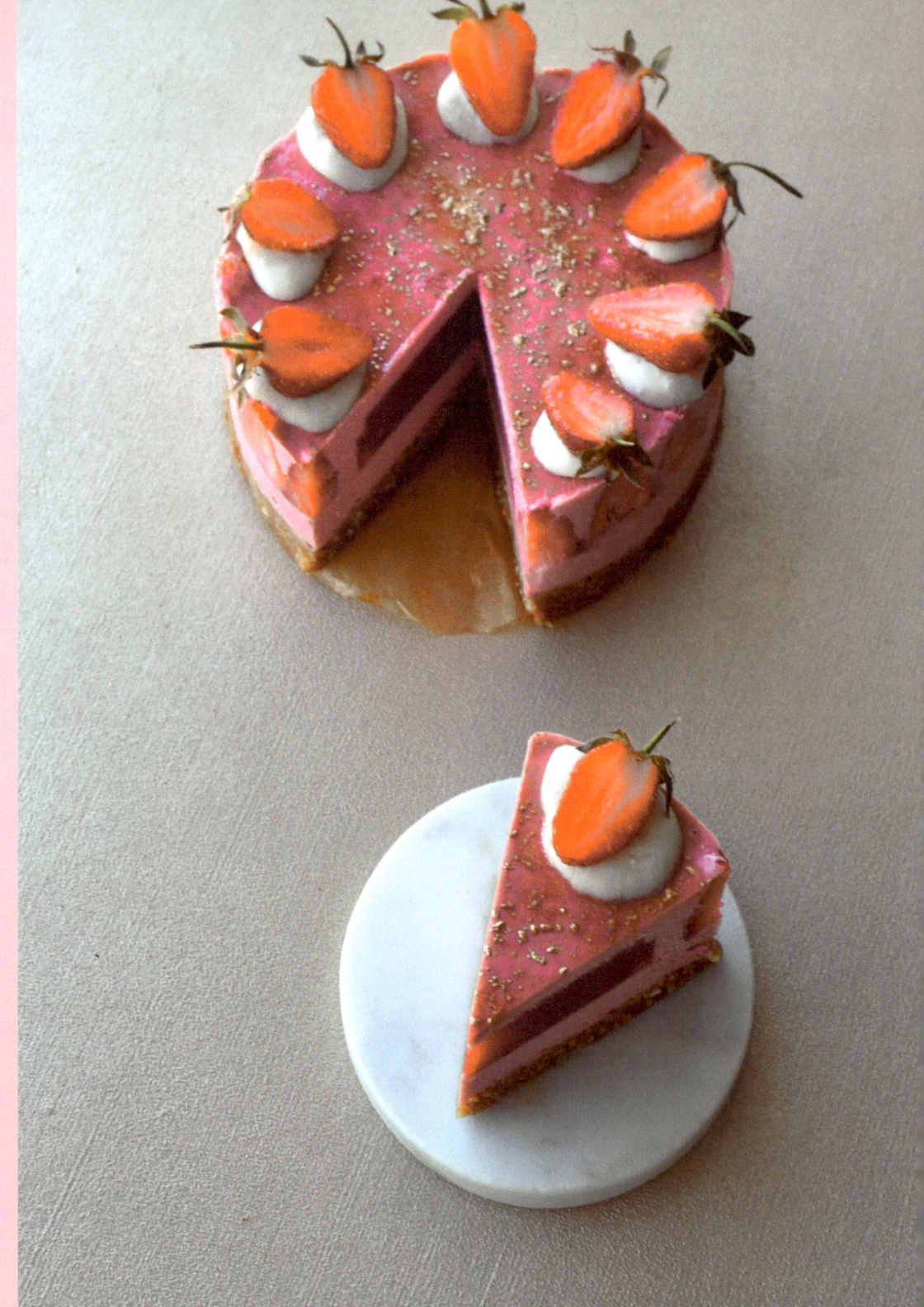

Summertime, the princess cake gets tough competition from the equally delicious strawberry cake (jordgubbstårta). This symbol of Swedish summer is often made at home, layering sponge cake, vanilla cream and strawberry jam (or mashed fresh strawberries and a pinch of sugar) and then covering the whole thing with whipped cream. On top, a generous cluster of fresh strawberries.

Time - 2 hours prep + 4 hours setting
Serves - 6-8

Crust

50 g coconut sugar powdered
50 g oat flour
50 g walnut flour
25 g desiccated coconut
25 ml maple syrup
25 ml virgin coconut oil melted
7.5 ml coconut aminos
15 ml coconut milk or water

Strawberry Cheesecake Filling

1 batch fermented cashew (page 29)
190 g coconut cream
40 g fresh beetroot
40 ml maple syrup
50 ml virgin coconut oil melted
30 ml lemon juice
15 g freeze dried strawberry powder
1 tsp vanilla extract

Strawberry Gel

170 ml fresh beetroot juice
60 g strawberry puree
30 ml maple syrup
150 g irish moss gel

Decoration

250 g coconut whipped cream
5-6 fresh strawberries halved
Edible gold powder

CRUST

Place oat flour, walnut flour, coconut sugar and desiccated coconut into your food processor. Mix together. Then add the maple syrup, coconut oil, coconut aminos or tamari. Process to combine together until the dough holds together. If it is dry, add 1 tbsp water or coconut milk, so the dough holds easily. Transfer dough in a 15 cm round cake mould lined parchment paper. Press down and flatten out with the back of a spoon. Keep in the refrigerator.

STRAWBERRY CHEESECAKE FILLING

Make a batch of fermented cashew cream according to instructions given on the page 31. Once prepared, place the fermented cashew cream in the blender, add the coconut cream, fresh beet juice, lemon juice and vanilla extract. Blend together until smooth. Then add the maple syrup, freeze dried strawberry powder and melted coconut oil. Continue to blend until you get a silky smooth unicorn color cream. Pour the half of the cream over the crust. Keep in the other half in the refrigerator. Transfer cake to the freezer for about 1-1.5 hours.

STRAWBERRY GEL

To make strawberry gel, place all the ingredients in the food processor. Blend until smooth puree. Let it sit for 10 minutes until it becomes gelly. It is thick but pourable at this point but will solidify when chilled. Transfer gel into a 10 cm round cake mould. Freeze for 2 hours.

ASSEMBLY

Once time is up, remove the strawberry gel from the mould.
Meanwhile, clean, dry and cut the strawberries in in half from top to bottom and arrange around the edge of the prepared tin, cut side-up.
Carefully place the strawberry gel in the middle of the cake. Then pour the rest of the strawberry cheesecake filling over the gel. Tap on counter carefully to remove air bubbles. Freeze for 4 hours. Decorate with coconut whipped cream and halved strawberries, dust some edible gold powder before serving.

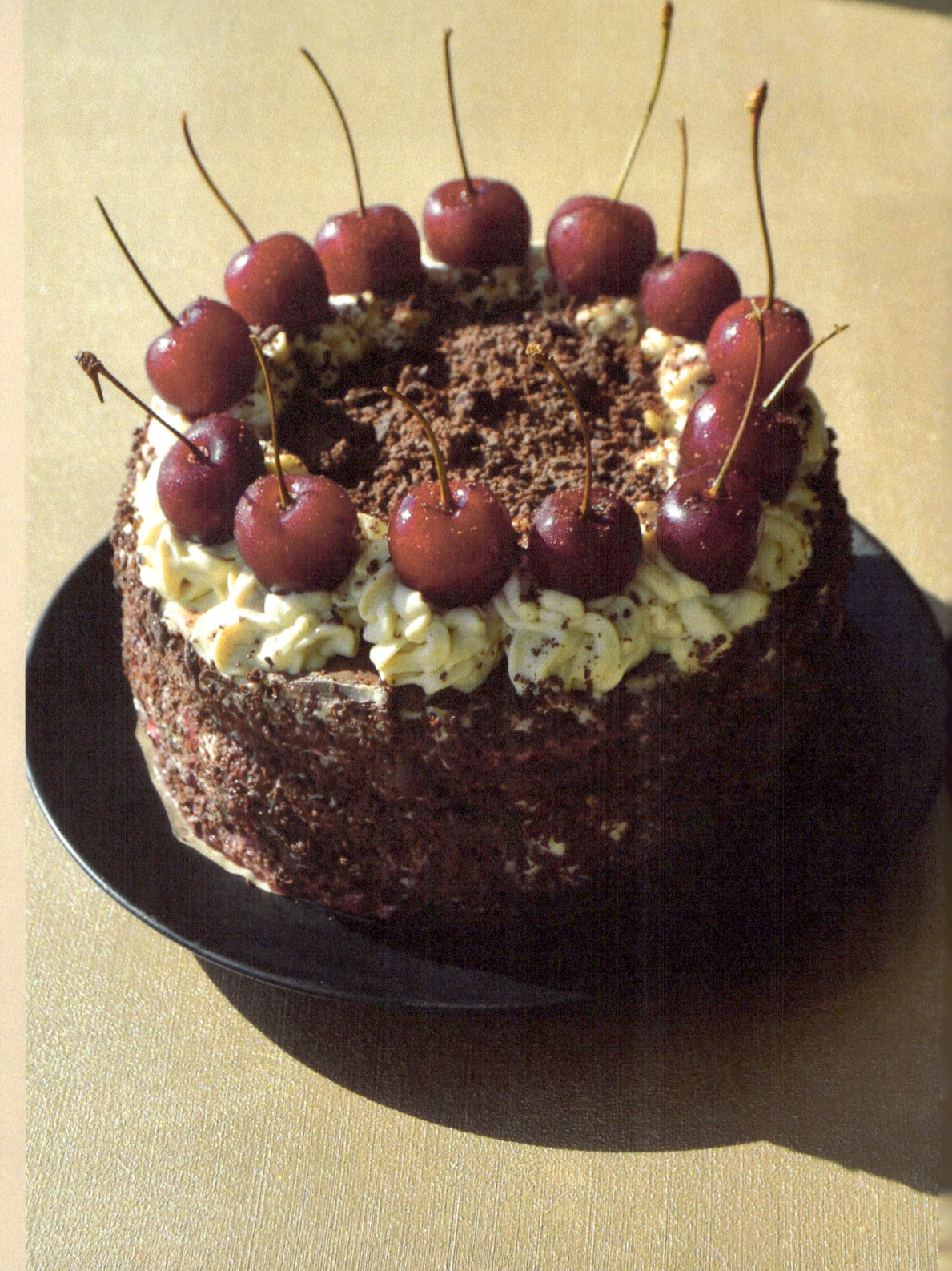

RAW FIKA

BLACK FOREST CAKE

Black Forest gâteau or Black Forest cake is a chocolate sponge cake with a rich cherry filling based on the German dessert Schwarzwälder Kirschtorte. It is not Swedish but internationally accepted and one of the most loved cakes. As it is one of my favorites, we wanted to include this recipe as well. The traditional version consists of multiple layers of chocolate sponge cake with whipped cream and cherries, covered on each side with whipped cream and shredded chocolate, as well as with cherries on top. The usage of whipped cream as an ingredient is also crucial for these cakes, giving them a light and fluffy structure. The aesthetic beauty of a black forest cake is almost always mentioned in the same breath as its rich and elegant taste. I believe you will love this raw version, which is very close to the original one.

Time - 3 hours prep + 6 hours setting
Serves - 6-8

Chocolate Crust
180 g almond flour
100 g coconut sugar powdered
40 g raw cacao powder
20 g almond butter
40 ml virgin coconut oil melted
30 ml tamari or coconut aminos
15 ml water as needed to bind
A pinch pink himalayan salt

Cashew Vanilla Cream
150 g raw cashews soaked
130 g coconut cream
35 ml virgin coconut oil melted
20 g cacao butter melted
65 ml coconut nectar syrup
15 ml lemon juice
1 tbsp vanilla extract
A pinch pink himalayan salt

Cherry Jam
400 g defrosted sour cherries
40 ml coconut nectar syrup
30 g chia seeds

Avocado Chocolate Frosting
130 g avocado meat
120 g coconut cream
30 g raw cacao powder
70 ml maple syrup
40 ml virgin coconut oil melted
20 g raw cacao butter melted
15 ml tamari or coconut aminos

Coconut Frosting
1 batch coconut frosting Page 26

Whipped Cream
250 ml coconut cream (thick part of the can)
35 g erythritol or monk fruit sweetener powdered
5 ml vanilla extract

Decoration
50 g shredded raw chocolate
13-14 fresh sour cherries

CHOCOLATE CRUST

Place almond flour, coconut sugar, cacao powder and salt into food processor. Mix together. Then add almond butter, melted coconut oil, vanilla extract, coconut aminos or tamari and water as needed. Process to combine together until dough comes together. Divide the dough into two. Line 2 X 15 cm round cake mold with parchment paper. Press down the dough into mold, flatten out with your hands and the back of spoon. Repeat the process for the other part of the dough in other 15 cm cake mold. Set the molds in the refrigerator while making the other components of the cake.

CHERRY JAM

Place defrosted cherries in a blender, add the coconut nectar, blend together. Transfer the mixture in a large container or bowl, add the chia seeds, stir well. Dehydrate in the food dehydrator at 46°C for 6 hours or overnight, until you get thick jam.

CASHEW VANILLA CREAM

Soak your cashews for 4-5 hours or overnight. Then rinse and dry. Place to your blender. Add the coconut cream, coconut nectar syrup, lemon juice vanilla and salt. Blend until smooth. Then add melted coconut oil and cacao butter. Process again until everything combined well and you have a silky smooth mixture.

AVOCADO CHOCOLATE

Place peeled and cored avocado in the food processor. Add coconut milk, maple syrup and tamari. Blend together. Then add cacao powder, melted coconut oil and coconut butter. Mix together until you get a silky smooth mixture.

COCONUT FROSTING

Make a batch of coconut frosting according to instructions given on the page 28. Freeze mixture overnight, and in the morning sit at room temperature for 1-2 hours or until it becomes creamy and ready to cover the cake and pipe.

DECORATION

Meanwhile, wash and dry your cherries, leave them with stems for decoration. Set aside.

Using a microplane, grate half of the chocolate in a bowl to use for covering the sides of your cake. Coating the sides of your cake is also a great way to conceal a not-so-perfect frosting job, and it adds dimension and fun to any cake.
Do not shred the rest of chocolate at this stage as we want to create dusting effect, we will shred it on the cake.

ASSEMBLY

Remove one of the crusts from the fridge. Pour the half of sour cherry jam on the crust. Spread evenly using a spatula or spoon. Freeze it for one hour. Once time is up, remove from the freezer, pour the half of cashew vanilla cream. Freeze for another hour. Once done, remove from the freezer, pour the half of avocado chocolate cream. Freeze again for 2 hours. Once done, remove from the cake from the freezer. Remove the second crust from the fridge and unmold, place it on the avocado layer. Gently press down so it holds the cream. Spread the rest of sour cherry jam over the crust. Freeze for one hour, then pour the rest of cashew vanilla cream.

After freezing it for one hour, lastly pour the avocado chocolate cream and freeze the whole cake for 3 hours.

Meanwhile, remove the coconut frosting from the freezer. Once it reaches to room temperature, start covering the cake. Spread the frosting to the edge of the layer with an offset spatula. Then, spread the frosting across the down the sides of the cake. It can help to spin the turntable slowly so you get even coverage. After covered your cake, leave the overlapping pieces of parchment paper under the cake and put some of the shredded chocolate in the palm of your hand. Fill your hand quite full so that you don't end up smudging the frosting with your hand. Gently pat the coating into the frosting. Working your way around the cake, pat the coating into the frosting. Don't press too hard—use just enough pressure to ensure the coating sticks to the frosting.

Brush off the excess coating. Use a pastry brush to brush off the excess coating. Gently pull away the parchment paper to reveal the beautiful finished cake.

To decorate the top of the cake, grip the microplane or other tool with one hand and the rest of chocolate in the other. Hold them over your dessert and run the chocolate along the microplane. This will create a dusting effect. Continue until you're satisfied with the amount of grated chocolate.

To make whipped coconut cream, before you start, make sure you are using a brand of coconut cream with a minimum 95% of coconut extract or 60% fat in the can. It is often referred to as full-fat coconut cream on the can. Place the can of coconut cream in the fridge overnight along with the bowl and whipping tools you will use to whip the cream. The next day, remove the can from the fridge, don't shake it. Open the can and carefully scoop out the thick hard part that appears on top of the can, making sure you leave all the water at the bottom of the can. Place the coconut cream, powder sweetener, and vanilla in the refrigerated bowl. Start whipping the cream at high speed with an electric mixter until it becomes light and fluffy like whipped cream. If it is not thick enough to pipe, just keep in the refrigerator for couple of hours before using.

Fill a piping bag with the whipped cream and choose a tip based on what design you want to make. To practice your piping skills, lay a piece of parchment paper on a baking sheet and try out different tips before you decorate the cake itself. Once you are ready, pipe the frosting to form a circular wreath as shown in the picture. Put cherries on the frostings.

Chill the cake at least 4 hours before cutting, so all the layers come to same temperature.

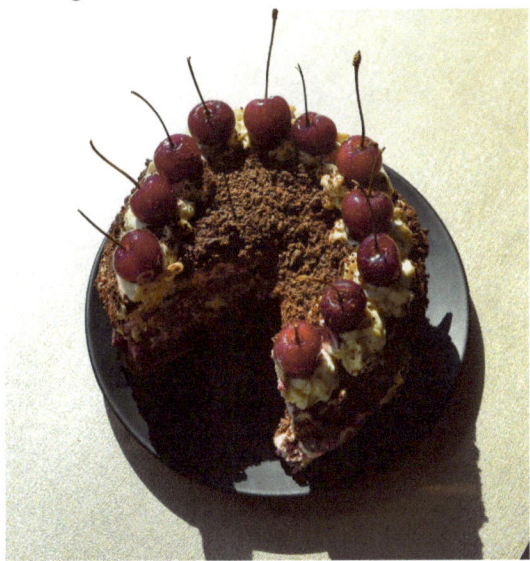

RAW FIKA

PEANUT PRALINE CAKE

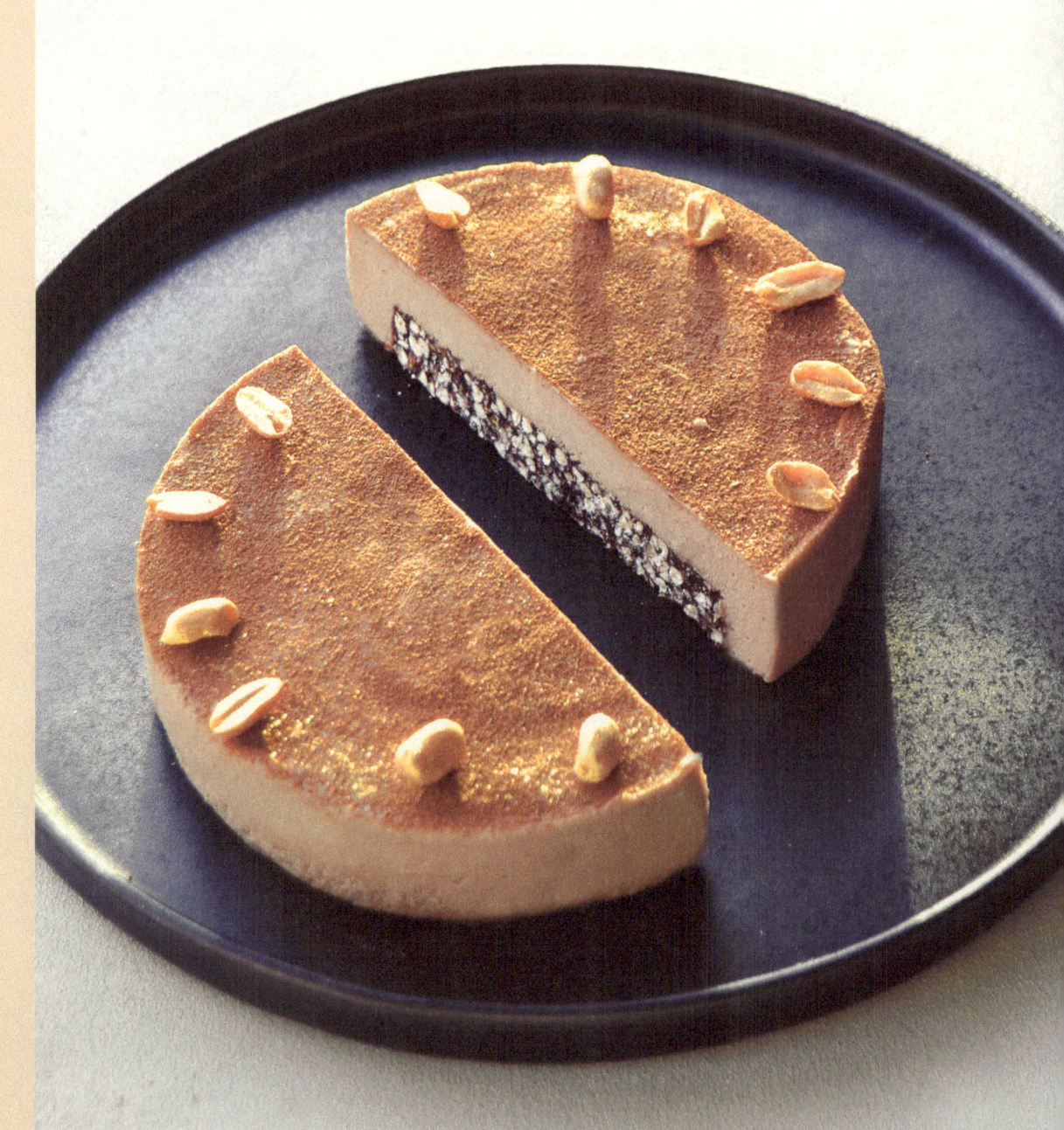

Time - 1 hour prep + 5 hours setting
Serves - 6-8

Crust
40 g dried raisins soaked
50 g buckini (activated dehydrated buckwheat groats)
20 ml maple syrup
10 g peanut butter
10 ml virgin coconut oil melted
7 g raw cacao powder
A pinch pink himalayan salt

Peanut Cream
95 g raw cashews soaked
95 g coconut cream
50 ml maple syrup
40 g peanut butter
10 g raw cacao powder
30 ml virgin coconut oil melted
20 g raw cacao butter melted
4 drops Medicine Flower's peanut flavor
A pinch of pink himalayan salt

Toppings
Cinnamon powder
Edible gold powder
Peanuts

CRUST
Soak your raisins in warm water for 5 minutes, then rinse and dry, add to a food processor. Add maple syrup, raw cacao powder, coconut oil, peanut butter and salt. Blend together. Lastly add buckini and stir to combine until buckinis covered with the mixture well. Transfer mixture in a 10 cm round mold lined parchment paper. Freeze while making the cream.

PEANUT CREAM
To make filling, place soaked rinsed cashews in a high speed blender, add coconut cream, maple syrup, peanut butter, cacao powder and salt. Blend until smooth. Lastly add melted coconut oil and cacao butter. Process again until silky smooth. Taste it, adjust the flavours, add more salt for a salty balanced taste or more maple syrup for a sweet finish.

ASSEMBLY
Remove the cake crust from the freezer. Unmould crust from 10 cm round tin, place in a 15 round cake mold with a bottom. Make sure crust is sitting in the middle of mold.

Then pour the cream over the crust. Gently tap the mold in order to prevent bubbles. Freeze at least 5 hours or overnight before cutting and serving.

Once your cake is ready, dust some cinnamon powder, edible gold powder. Decorate with peanuts.

RAW FIKA

TIRAMISU CAKE

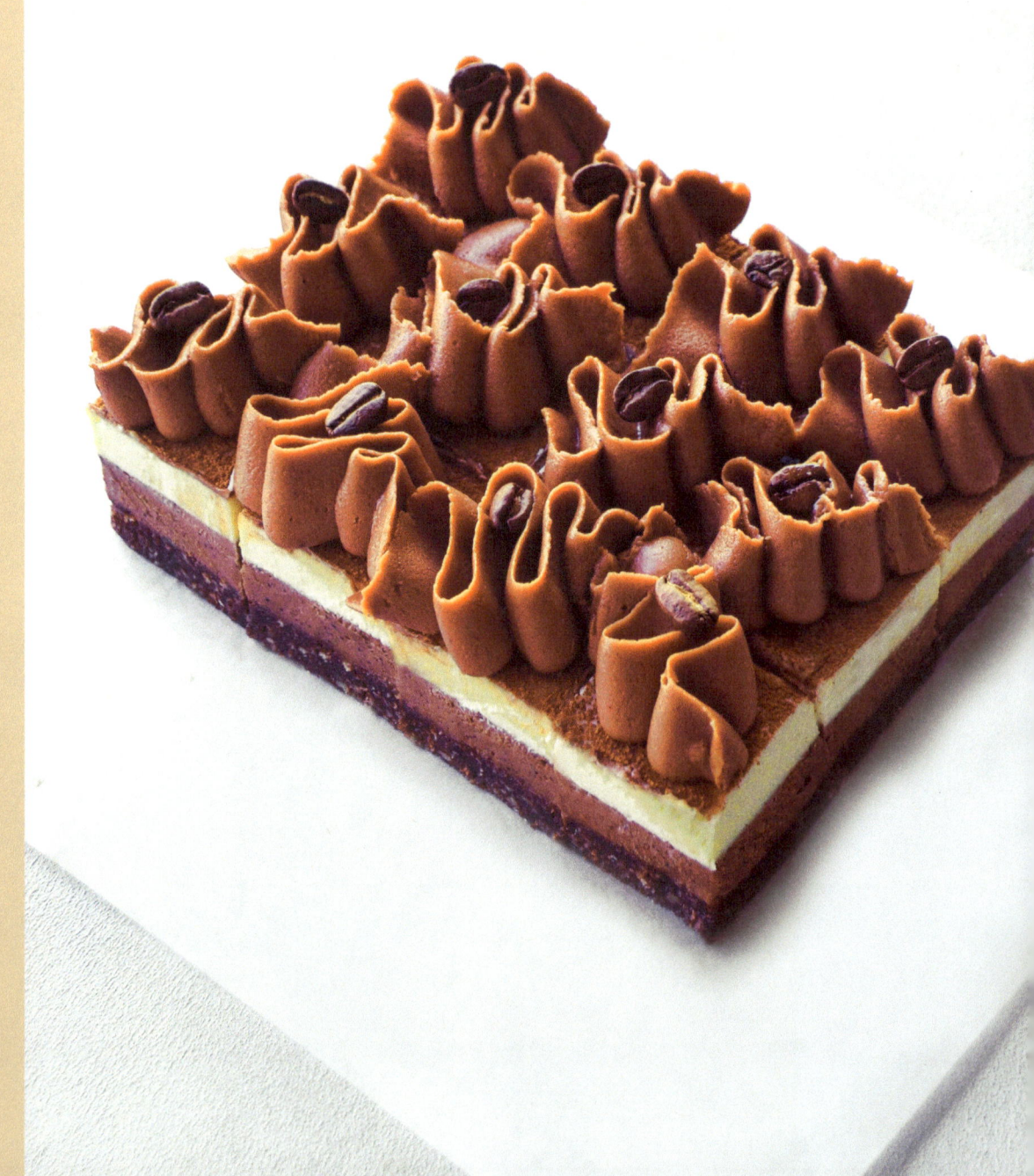

Time - 2 hours prep + 6 hours setting
Serves - 12

Crust
85 g raw walnuts
90 g medjool dates soaked
15 g desiccated coconut
15 g raw cacao powder
30 ml espresso freshly brewed
15 ml virgin coconut oil melted
7 g ground coffee beans
1/8 tsp pink himalayan salt

Coffee Mousse
75 g raw cashews soaked
110 g coconut cream
50 g medjool dates soaked
35 ml virgin coconut oil melted
15 g ground coffee beans
30 ml maple syrup
45 g irish moss paste
15 g raw cacao powder
1/4 tsp pink himalayan salt

Coconut Mascarpone
75 g young coconut meat
100 g coconut cream
60 g irish moss paste
35 ml maple syrup
22 ml virgin coconut oil melted
18 g cacao butter melted
7 ml lemon juice
1/4 tsp pink himalayan salt

Decoration
1 batch avocado chocolate frosting (page 41) + coffee beans to decorate.

CRUST
To make crust, place walnuts, desiccated coconut, cacao powder, ground coffee beans and salt in a food processor, mix together to combine. Then add medjool dates, freshly brewed espresso and coconut oil. Process again until dough comes together. Transfer dough to a 15x15 cm square mold. Press down with your hands and then with the back of a spoon. Flatten out as much as possible. Let it sit in the fridge while making the coffee mousse.

COFFEE MOUSSE
To make coffee mousse, place soaked, rinsed raw cashews to a high speed blender. Add coconut cream, medjool dates, ground coffee beans, maple, irish moss paste, raw cacao powder and salt. Blend until you get a pretty smooth mixture. Lastly add melted coconut oil and blend again until well incomparated. Pour the mixture over the crust. Let it sit in the freezer for at least one hour in order to prevent mixing layers.

COCONUT MASCARPONE
To make coconut mascarpone, place the young coconut meat in a high speed blender, add the coconut cream, irish moss paste, maple syrup, lemon juice and salt. Blend everything until smooth.
Then add the melted coconut oil and cacao butter. Blend again until well incomparated.

ASSEMBLY
Remove the cake from the freezer, the coffee mousse should be firm enough when you touch with your fingers. Once it is cooled enough, pour the coconut mascarpone over the coffee mousse. Tap the mold in order to prevent bubbles. Freeze at least 4-5 hours before cutting. Unmould the tiramisu, using a ruler cut into equal squares. Make the avocado frosting according to the instructions on the page 41. Transfer the cream in a piping bag with Wilton 125 tip. Pipe the cream on the squares. Place coffee bean on each square. Dust some cacao powder and edible gold powder if desired.

CHOCOLATE HAZELNUT CAKE

RAW FIKA

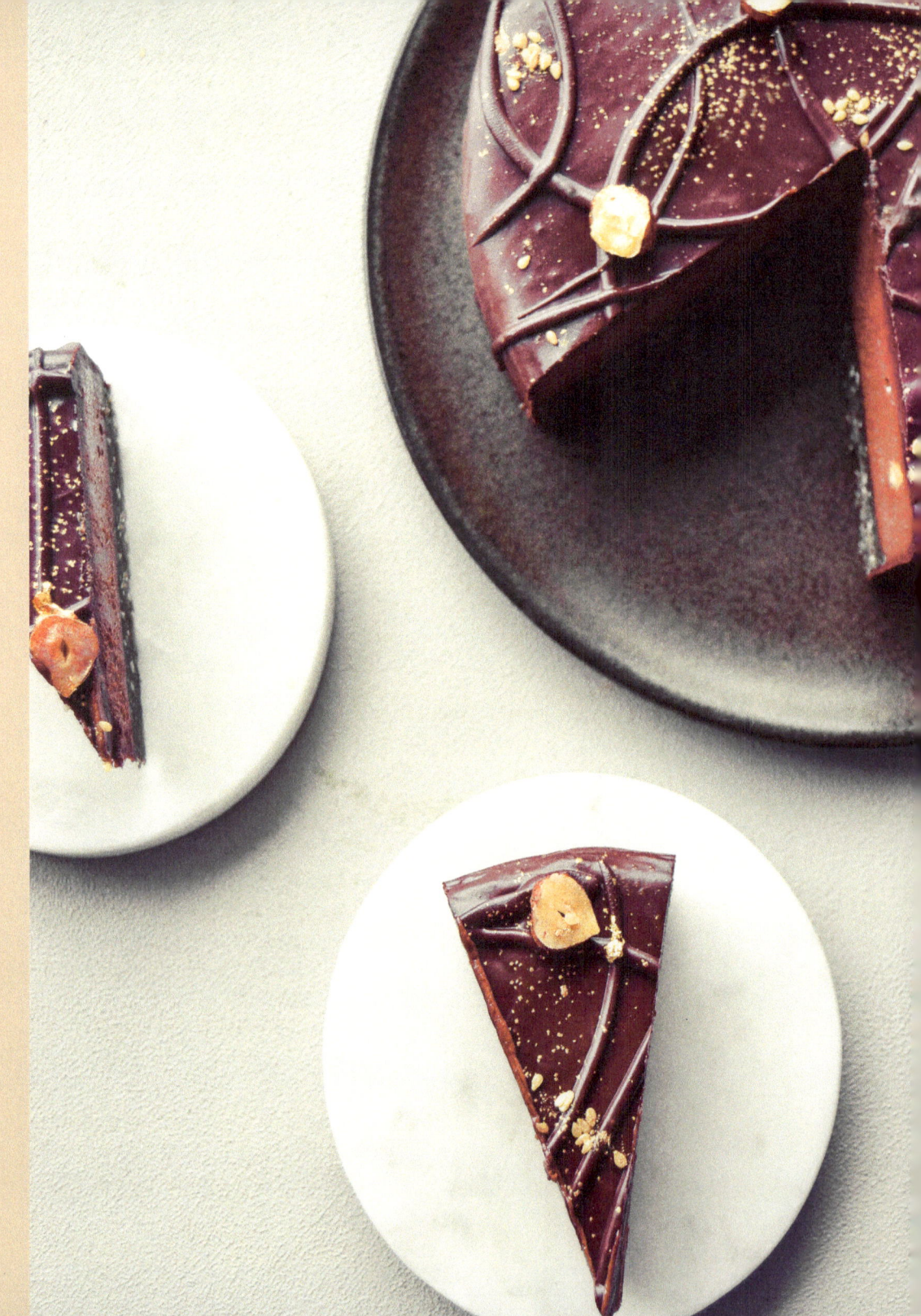

Time - 2 hours + 4 hours setting
Serves - 6 slices

Crust
80 g activated dehydrated hazelnut flour
30 g activated dehydrated buckwheat groats
25 g coconut sugar powdered
15 ml maple syrup
10 g raw cacao powder
40 g virgin coconut oil melted
15 ml coconut milk
1/4 tsp charcoal powder
1/8 tsp ground coffee beans
1/8 tsp pink himalayan salt

Chocolate Cream
100 g cashews soaked
50 g hazelnut butter unroasted
55 g freshly brewed espresso
20 g raw cacao powder
30 g hazelnut milk
60 ml maple syrup
45 ml virgin coconut oil melted
7 ml lemon juice
1/4 tsp pink himalayan salt

Chocolate Ganache
70 g raw chocolate melted (53% cacao mass)
63 g coconut cream
8 ml virgin coconut oil melted

Decoration
Halved hazelnuts
Edible gold powder

CRUST
Place the hazelnut flour, buckwheat groats, coconut sugar, cacao powder, ground coffee beans and salt into your food processor. Process to get a coarse flour. Then add the coconut milk and melted coconut oil. Process again until dough comes together.
Line a 15 cm round cake mould with parchment paper. Press the dough firmly with your fingers first, then flatten with the back of a spoon. Set aside while you are making the chocolate cream.

CHOCOLATE CREAM
Place the cashews, espresso, hazelnut milk, maple, lemon juice and salt into your blender. Process until you get a silky smooth mixture. Then add the melted coconut oil, hazelnut butter and cacao powder. Blend again until incorparated well.
Pour the chocolate cream into the cake crust. Chill the cake in the freezer for 6-7 hours or overnight.

CHOCOLATE GANACHE
Melt the raw chocolate using bain marie, add the coconut cream and coconut oil, then mix together until incorparated well. Then use an electric whisk to whip the chocolate ganache for a couple of minutes. Let it cool at room temperature for 15-20 minutes. Chocolate ganache shouldn't be warm but still liquid enough for the next step, so allow it to come to room temperature.

ASSEMBLY
Once you removed the cake from the freezer, set aside 2 tbsp of the ganache to use for decoration later, then pour the ganache over the cake, put it back in the fridge for at least 1 hour. Place the ganache in a piping bag and cut a very small tip off the end. Pipe stripes of chocolate on top of cake. Garnish with halved hazelnuts and gold leaf. Dust some gold powder if desired. Chill for 30 minutes.
Once you removed the cake from the freezer, allow it to sit in the fridge for 1-2 hours before slicing it smoothly.

BROWNIE WITH CHOCOLATE GANACHE & RASPBERRIES

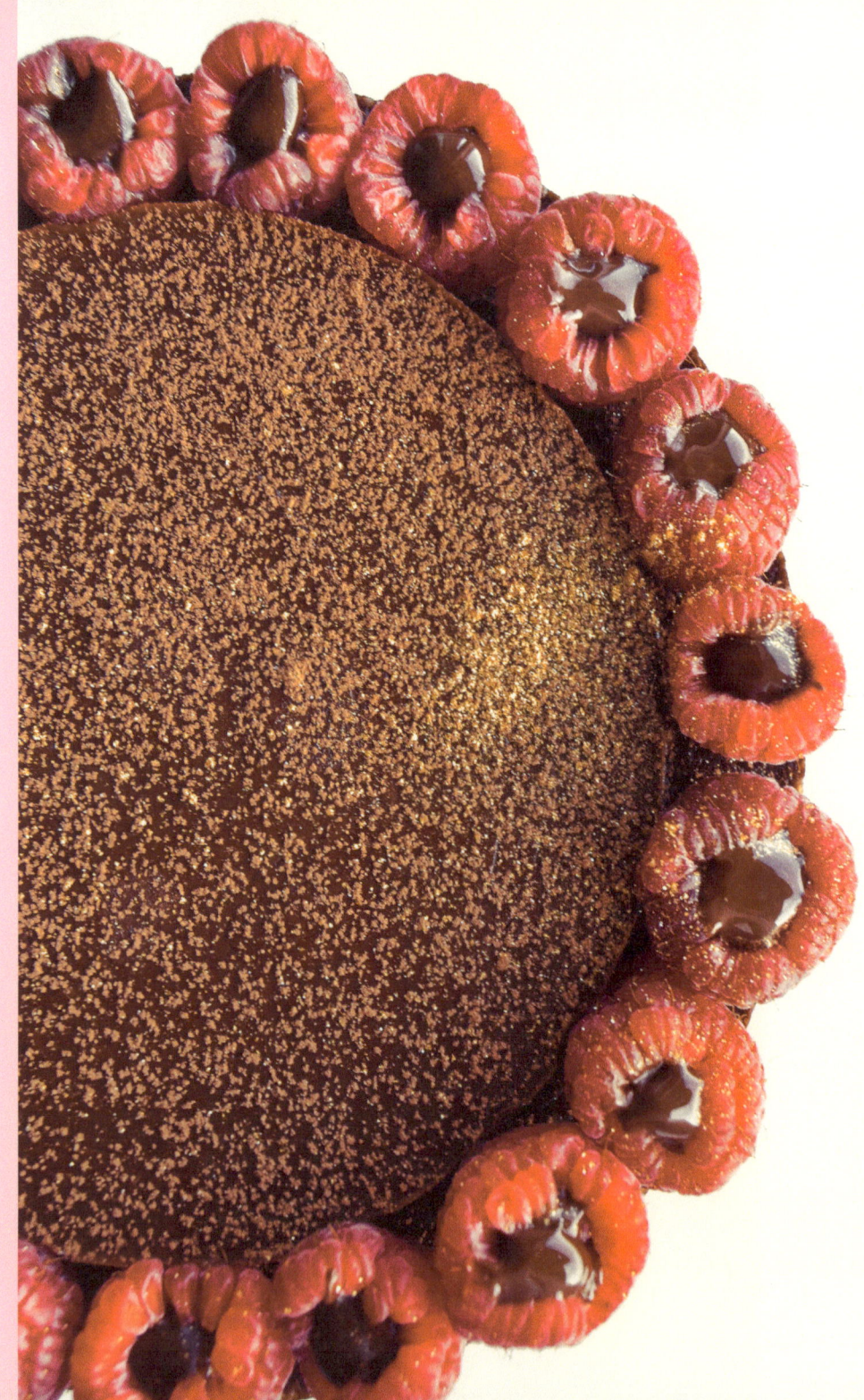

Time - 10 min prep + 45 min setting
Serves - 15 cm round cake mold, 15 very thin slices

Crust
50 g oat flour
50 g almond flour
50 g buckini
20 g cacao powder
10 g coconut sugar powdered
40 ml maple syrup
40 ml virgin coconut oil
5 ml tamari
A pinch pink himalayan salt

Praline Ganache
60 g raw chocolate melted
70 g almond butter
5 g miso paste
15 ml virgin coconut oil melted
A pinch pink himalayan salt

Garnish
125 g fresh raspberries
35 g raw chocolate melted
7 ml virgin coconut oil melted
A pinch pink himalayan salt
Edible gold powder
Raw cacao powder

CRUST
Place oat flour, almond flour, cacao powder, coconut sugar and salt into your food processor, combine together. Then add maple syrup, tamari and coconut oil. Combine together until dough comes together. Lastly add buckini and blend again. We want some crispy elements in the dough, so do not overdo your food processor, just pulse a few times. Once done, remove from the food processor. Line a 15 cm round cake mold with parchment paper, transfer dough to the mold. Press down and flatten out as much as possible.

PRALINE GANACHE
To make ganache, melt your raw chocolate using bain marie, add almond butter, miso paste, coconut oil and salt. Mix together until everything combined well.

ASSEMBLY
Place a 10 cm round cake ring in the middle of 15 cm cake mold with the cake crust you have recently made. Pour the ganache in the middle of 10 cm ring. Immediately freeze for 1 hour.
Once time is up, remove from the freezer, unmold the cake. Dust some raw cacao and edible gold powder.
Start arranging the raspberries, place them around the cake.
Melt raw chocolate using bain marie, add coconut oil and salt. Whisk well. Let it cool at least 20 minutes at room temperature. Then transfer to a piping bag. Cut the end very small. Fill the raspberries with chocolate. Thinly slice the cake and serve.

RAW FIKA

EMERALD PANDAN
CHEESECAKE

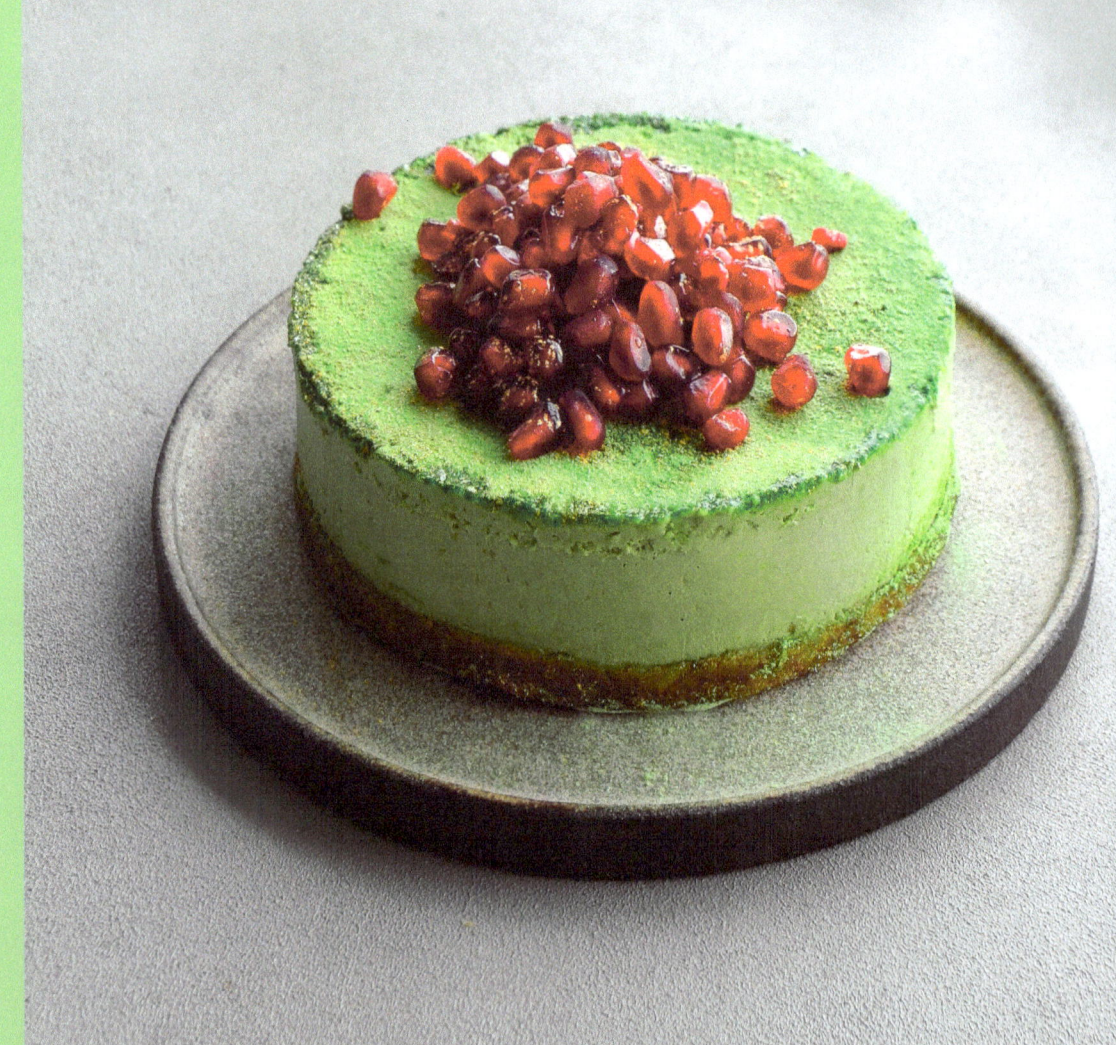

Time - 40 minutes prep + 3 hrs setting
Serves - 6 slices

Macadamia Crust
60 g macadamia flour
20 g macadamia butter
60 g dried mango soaked
15 ml maple syrup
10 g cacao butter melted
15 g desiccated coconut
7 ml coconut aminos

Emerald Pandan Cream
150 g macadamia soaked
90 g coconut cream
60 ml coconut water
45 ml lime juice
50 ml maple syrup
25 g cacao butter melted
25 g pandan powder + more for dusting

Decoration
Pandan powder to sprinkle
Pomegranate seeds to serve

MACADAMIA CRUST
Place macadamia flour, soaked rinsed mango, macadamia butter, maple syrup, desiccated coconut and coconut aminos in a food processor. Mix together. Lastly add melted coconut butter, process again.
Transfer dough in a 15 cm round cake tin lined parchment paper. Press down with your hands and flatten out with the back of a spoon. Freeze while making the cream.

EMERALD PANDAN CREAM
Place soaked rinsed macadamias in the blender. Add the coconut cream, coconut water, lime juice, maple, pandan powder and salt. Blend until smooth. Add melted cacao butter and process again until you get a silky smooth cream.

ASSEMBLY
Remove the crust from the freezer. Pour the emerald pandan cream over the macadamia crust. Gently tap the mold to prevent bubbles.
Freeze the cake for 3 hours. Once cooled enough, unmold, dust some pandan powder. Place pomegranate seeds on top or decorate how you like. Slice and serve.

RAW FIKA

MANGO GOLDEN MILK CHEESECAKE

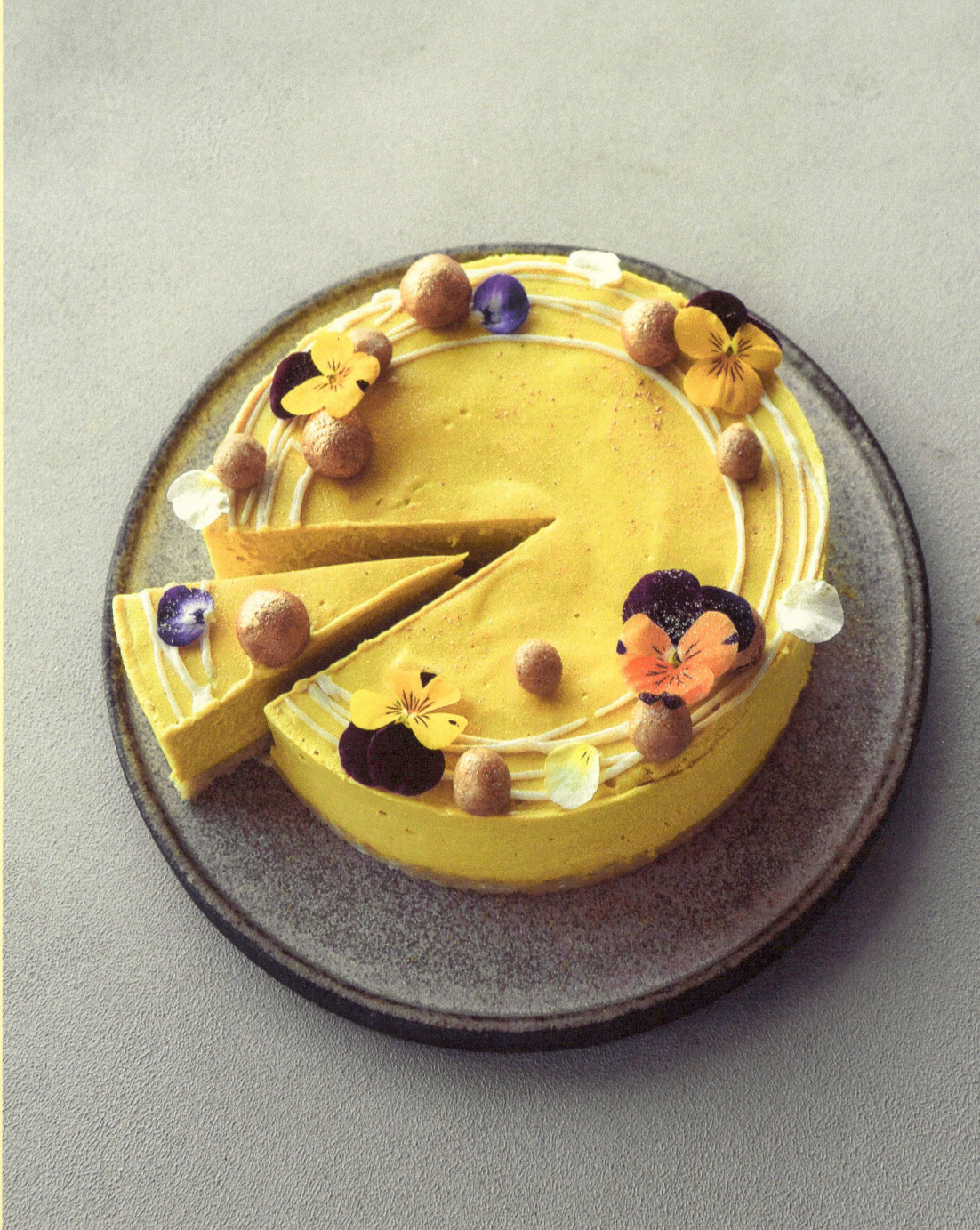

Time - 1 hour + 4 hours setting
Serves - 6 slices

Crust
50 g macadamia flour
30 g desiccated coconut
20 g macadamia butter
15 ml virgin coconut oil melted
35 ml maple syrup
A pinch pink himalayan salt

Golden Milk Mango Cream
140 g raw cashews soaked
75 g fresh mango meat
70 g coconut cream
45 ml maple syrup
45 ml lemon juice
45 ml raw cacao butter melted
15 ml virgin coconut oil melted
5 g turmeric powder
A pinch pink himalayan salt

Cookie Balls
55 g macadamia butter
15 g coconut flour
20 g coconut sugar powdered
5 g cacao butter melted
A pinch pink himalayan salt
Edible gold powder

Coconut Glaze
50 g young coconut meat
20 ml coconut milk
25 ml maple syrup
30 ml virgin coconut oil melted
5 ml lemon juice

CRUST
Place the macadamia flour, salt and desiccated coconut into your food processor, process together. Then add the macadamia butter, coconut oil and maple syrup. Process again until it comes together. Line a 15 cm round cake mold with parchment paper. Transfer dough to your mold. Press down with your fingers then with a back of spoon. Flatten out as much as possible. Set in the fridge while making cream.

GOLDEN MILK MANGO CREAM
Place mango, cashews, coconut cream, maple, lemon juice, salt and turmeric into your blender. Blend on high speed until you get silky smooth mixture. Then add melted coconut oil and coconut butter. Blend again until incomparated well. Pour mixture over the crust. Place in the freezer for at least 4 hours before unmoulding.

COOKIE BALLS
In a small bowl, mix all the cookie ball ingredients together. The dough should come together when you press with your fingers but still soft to form in a ball. Chill for 25-30 minutes. Then make small balls with your hands. Roll into edible gold powder if desired. Set in the fridge before decorate the cake.

COCONUT GLAZE
To make coconut glaze, place all coconut glaze ingredients to your blender. Blend on high speed until silky smooth. Transfer mixture in a piping bag. If it is too runny, just sit it in the fridge for 10-15 minutes. Then cut a very small tip off the end of piping bag.

ASSEMBLY
Remove the cake from the freezer, unmould. Pipe circles with coconut glaze on the cake. Keep the rest of your glaze in the freezer to use later in cake decorations. It will keep up to 2 months. Place some cookie balls around the circle. Decorate with pansies. Dust some edible glitter. Slice and serve.

RAW FIKA

CHERRY BUCKWHEAT CAKE BARS

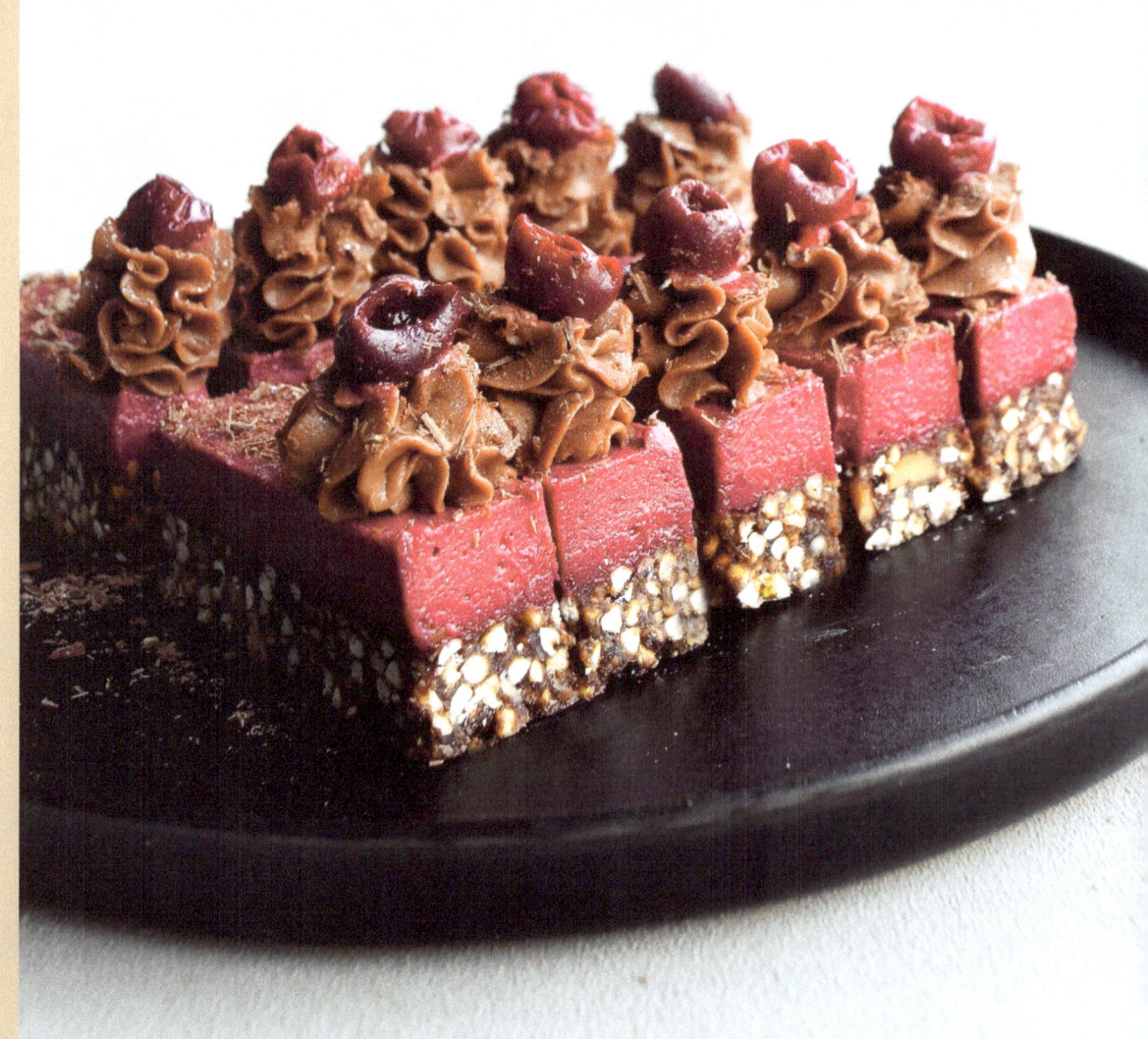

Time - 2 hours + 4 hours setting
Serves - 12

Buckwheat Cereal
150 g buckwheat activated dehydrated
50 ml maple syrup
30 g peanuts
10 g coconut sugar
10 g cacao powder
1/8 tsp pink himalayan salt

Cereal Crust
65 g medjool dates pitted
30 g macadamia butter
10 ml virgin coconut oil melted
15 g cacao butter melted
1 batch buckwheat cereal

Cherry Compote
100 g frozen pitted cherries
30 g coconut sugar or monk fruit sweetener powdered
A pinch pink himalayan salt

Cherry Filling
85 g cashews soaked
65 g coconut cream
50 ml coconut nectar syrup
1 batch cherry compote
5 g beetroot powder
20 ml virgin coconut oil melted
10 g cacao butter melted
15 ml lemon juice
A pinch pink himalayan salt

BUCKWHEAT CEREAL
Soak raw buckwheat groats in warm water for 30-40 minutes, then rinse well. Transfer to a mixing bowl. Add maple syrup, peanuts, coconut sugar, cacao powder and salt. Mix everything until combined well. Transfer to a dehydrator sheet lined parchment paper. Dehydrate at 42°C for 4-5 hours. It must be completely dried. You may need to flip the groats after 2 hours.

CEREAL CRUST
Once buckwheat cereal is dried, transfer to the food processor, add the medjool dates, macadamia butter and melted cacao butter. Process until dough comes together.
Transfer the cereal into a 15x15 cm square cake mould lined parchment paper. Press with your fingers and then with a back of spoon. Flatten the dough out as much as possible. Keep in the fridge while you are making the cherry filling.

CHERRY COMPOTE
Place the defrosted cherries in a bowl. Add the coconut sugar and salt. Stir well. Dehydrate at 42°C for 6-8 hours or overnight until you get a thick jam-like consistency.

CHERRY FILLING
Place the cherry compote into blender, add cashews, coconut cream, coconut milk, coconut nectar syrup, beet powder, lemon juice and salt. Blend together until smooth. Then add melted coconut oil and coconut butter. Blend until everything combined well and you have a smooth mixture.

(continuted on the next page)

Chocolate Frosting

100 g cashews soaked
22 g coconut sugar powdered
15 g raw cacao powder
60 ml coconut milk
50 g coconut cream
7 m lemon juice
70 ml virgin coconut oil melted
1/8 tsp pink himalayan salt

Decoration

100 g dehydrated or fresh cherries
50 g shredded raw chocolate

CHOCOLATE FROSTING

To make chocolate frosting, place the soaked, rinsed cashews in a high speed blender. Add the coconut sugar (grind in coffee grinder beforehand), raw cacao powder, coconut milk and coconut cream, lemon juice and salt. Blend until you get a silky smooth mixture.
Then add the melted coconut oil, blend again until incomparated well. Place the cream in an airtight container and freeze at least 6 hours or overnight.

ASSEMBLY

Transfer cherry filling on the cereal crust. Tap the mould to remove bubbles. Freeze for 4-5 hours. Once done, unmould and slice into bars or squares.
In the morning, remove from the freezer, allow it to melt a bit at room temperature for about 1-1.5 hours you can place it in a dehydrator at 30°C for 30-40 minutes. Once the cream is set, transfer it to a desired piping bag, pipe the frosting on the top of cake slices. Place fresh or dehydrated cherries on the top of cream.
Shred some raw chocolate over the cakes. Serve immediately or keep in the refrigerator up to 4 days or in the freezer for 1-2 months.

ORANGE FLAVORED ALMOND CHOCO FUDGE

Time - 15 minutes prep + 3 hrs setting
Serves - 18 small squares

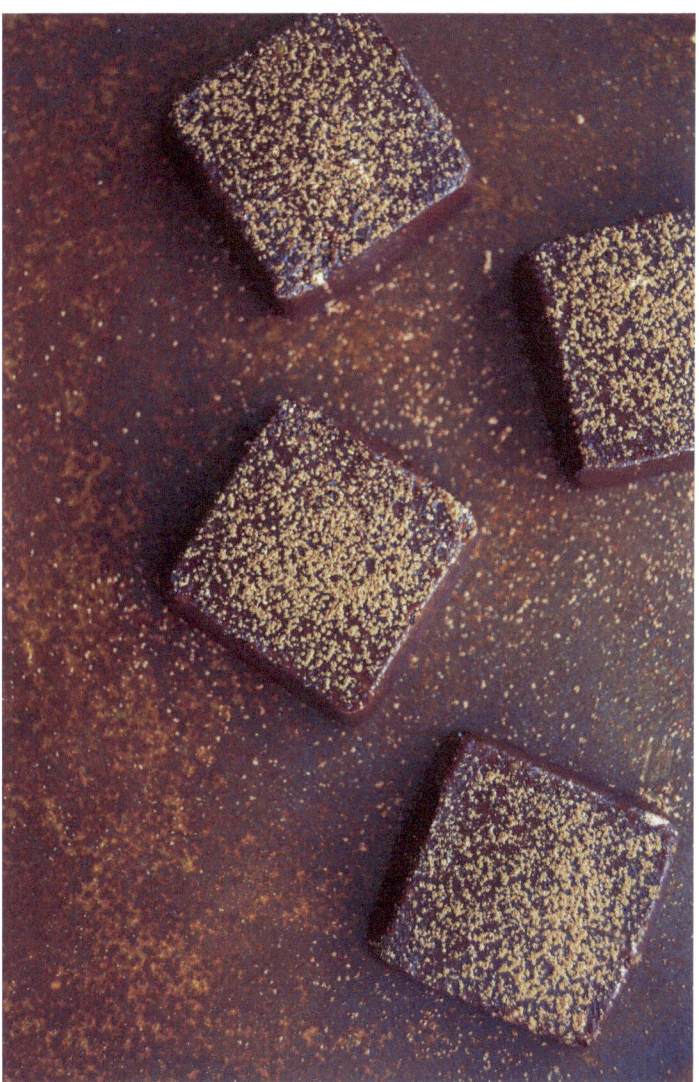

Ingredients

120 g almond butter
60 ml maple syrup
7 g raw cacao powder
75 ml melted cacao butter
4-5 drops orange essential oil

INSTRUCTIONS

Line a small 7x4 cm pan with parchment paper. Use a smaller dish if you prefer thicker fudge cubes or a larger one for thinner fudge bites.

In a small bowl, combine the almond butter, maple syrup, and raw cacao powder. Add the melted cacao butter, and orange essential oil if using, and whisk slowly until everything is smooth and fully combined. At first, cacao butter will stay on top but as you mix, it will start to combine with the other ingredients.

Once fully smooth, pour the fudge into the prepared dish and refrigerate at least 3 hours, or until firm. Using a hot knife, cut into 15 or 18 squares.

It will keep in the refrigerator for up to two weeks, or in the freezer for up to 3 months.

ORANGE FLAVORED TRUFFLES WITH CELERIAC CRUMB

Time - 30 min prep + 6 hours dehydration + 50 minutes setting
Serves - 8 balls

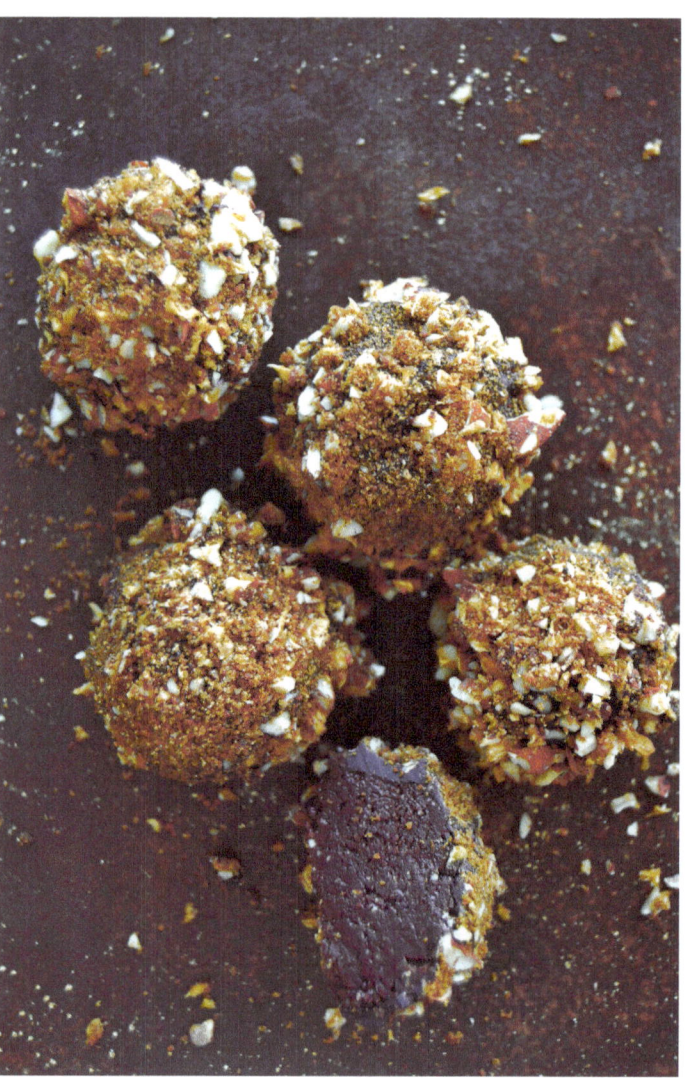

Ingredients

100 g almond butter
60 g raw chocolate melted
30 ml maple syrup
15 ml virgin coconut oil
A pinch of pink himalayan salt
5 drops wild orange essential oil

Topping

200 g celeriac
50 g almonds
4 tbsp coconut sugar
7-8 drops orange essential oil
100 g melted raw chocolate

INSTRUCTIONS

Make the topping according to instructions give on the page 43 (celeriac almond crumb).

In a blender, mix all ingredients until smooth. Transfer to a bowl, freeze for 45-50 minutes. Once cooled enough, it will be easier to shape the dough into small doughs with your hands. Make small balls for about 10-12. Place in the fridge.

Melt raw chocolate using bain marie, Dip the balls in the chocolate and then roll in celeriac topping. Refrigerate for 20 minutes.

ORANGE FLAVORED TOSCA COINS WITH CARAMEL

Time - 30 min prep
Serves - 12 pieces

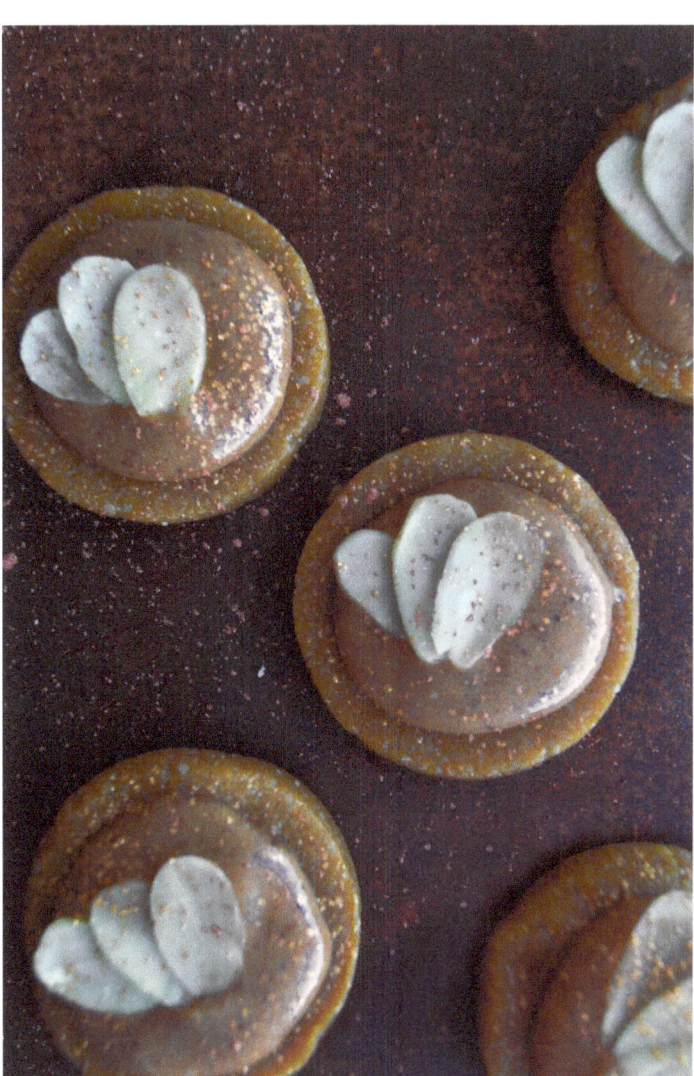

Ingredients

160 g almond flour
30 g coconut flour
80 ml maple syrup
30 ml virgin coconut oil melted
5-6 drops orange essential oil
1/2 tsp cinnamon
1/4 tsp cardamom
A pinch of pink himalayan salt

Mix all ingredients in a food processor. Divide into 12 pieces, make balls and press down with a cookie handle.

Caramel

70 g medjool dates soaked
40 ml coconut milk
25 ml virgin coconut oil melted
40 g almond butter
15 g lucuma powder
30 ml maple syrup
15 ml coconut aminos
1/8 tsp cinnamon powder
A pinch pink himalayan salt

In a blender, mix all ingredients until smooth. Drop a tablespoon caramel on the top of coins. Decorate with sliced almonds.

INDEX

A

almonds
- almond celeriac crumb — 32
- almond butter filling — 43
- almonds candied — 75
- almond marzipan — 35, 49, 50, 69

activated dehydrated nuts — 59
agave — 16
apples
- apple crumble pie — 46-47

arrack
- arrack extract — 13
- dammsugare with arrack — 47

avocado
- avocado chocolate frosting — 28, 41, 89, 92-93, 117
- avocado pistachio pandan — 98-99-100

B

brownie
- brownie coconut bacon — 56-57
- Swedish sticky brownie — 64-65
- brownie with hazelnut cream, avocado frosting & wakame crisp — 92-93

before you get started — 12
buckini — 17
- buckini crust — 115, 121, 127
- buckini cereal — 127

butterfly pea powder — 23
beetroot — 23
blender — 24
blueberry
- blueberry cake — 60-61-62-63
- bluberry chocolate brownie — 90-91

black forest
- black forest cake — 110, 111, 112, 113
- black forest roll — 78-79

C

cacao
- cacao powder — 14
- cacao mass — 14
- cacao nibs — 14
- cacao butter — 14

cake molds — 25
carrot cake — 34-35
coconut
- coconut bacon — 14
- coconut butter — 15
- coconut cream — 27
- coconut frosting — 26
- coconut oil — 15
- coconut sugar — 21
- coconut nectar syrup — 20
- coconut meat — 27
- coconut milk canned — 27
- coconut shredded — 27
- coconut bacon — 57
- coconut mascarpone — 117
- coconut pastry cream — 95-96
- coconut framboise cream — 98-99-100
- coconut crisp cookies — 102
- coconut glaze — 125

chocolate — 28
- chocolate base — 26
- chocolate frosting dark — 26
- chocolate frosting white — 40, 41
- chocolate ball semla — 52-53
- chocolate cookies — 65
- chocolate sauce — 82-83
- chocolate orange squares — 104-105
- choco ganache white — 107
- chocolate hazelnut cake — 118-119
- chocolate ganache — 119

coffee
- coffee grinder — 65
- coffee mousse (tiramisu) — 117
- coffee orange bars — 104-105

chokladbollar
chia seeds — 72-73
cashews — 18
chunky monkey icecream — 24
cheeseboard cookies — 65
cookie base — 70-71
cookie balls — 61
cherry — 125
- cherry buckwheat cake
- cherry compote — 126-127-128
- cherry jam — 127
  39, 79, 89, 111, 112

D

dates — 21
- date caramel — 31

dehydrated
- dehydrated cookie base — 30, 91
- dehydrated pastry — 79

dark chocolate frosting — 26
double boiler — 25
dammsugare
- green dammsugare — 48-49
- citron dammsugare — 50
- bounty dammsugare — 51

E

equipments	24-25
essential oils	22
extracts	22
erythritol	21, 45

F

fermented	
fermented cashew cream	29, 61, 109
fruit jams	29
blueberry jam	61, 91
cherry jam	39, 79, 89, 111, 112
raspberry jam	45, 67, 95, 96
food processor	24
food dehydrator	24
flavours and extracts	22
flaxseeds	18
fluffy cream buns	103

G

gojiberries	23

H

hibiscus	23
hemp seeds	19
hallongrottor	76-77

I

intro	6-7

J

japanese matcha yuzu cakes	106-107
jam	
blueberry jam	61, 91
cherry jam	39, 79, 89, 11, 112
raspberry jam	45, 67, 95, 96

K

kitkat praline cake	36-37
kanelbulle	
kanelbulle with chocolate	54-55
kanelbulle with caramel	42-43
kladdkaka	64-65, 85

L

lucia buns -lussekatter	80, 81

M

make-ahead fika staples	26
measuring spoons	25
matcha powder	23
matcha yuzu cream	107
macadamia	19
macadamia crust	123
maca powder	18
most common used dehydrated items	16
maple syrup	20
marzipan	
marzipan carrots	35
marzipan roses	69
green marzipan	49, 69
citron marzipan	50
strawberry marzipan	69

mascarpone	
coconut mascarpone	117
oat mascarpone	85
mango	
mango chocolate tart	88-89
mango golden milk cake	124-125
midsummer cake	108-109
mushroom wakame crisp	93

N

natural colorings	23
nut butters	30

O

olive oil extra virgin	15
oat mascarpone	85
orange	
orange coffee flavoured cake bars	104-105
orange flavoured almond choco fudge	129
orange flavoured truffles with celeriac crumb	130
orange flavoured tosca coins with caramel	131

P

pastry bag & piping set	25
pandan powder	23
pandan avocado pistachio framboise cake	98-99-100
emerald pandan cake	122, 123
pitaya powder	23
pine nuts	19
	79
pine cream	
praline	36-37
praline bars	107
macamia praline	114-115
peanut praline cake	121
praline ganache	66-67
princess cake	74-75
pepparkaksbollar	
pastry calender	8-11
porridge	101

R

raisins	21
raspberry	
raspberry caves	76-77
raspberry valentines day cake	94-95-96-97
raw fika recipes	33
ruler	25

S

sesame oil	15
scaler	25
Swedish items	13
sprouted	
sprouted whole oats	16
sprouted buckwheat (buckini)	17
spirulina powder	23
spice grinder	24
sunflower	
sunflower lecithin	22
sunflower cheese frosting	35
singoalla	38-39
semla	
chocolate ball semla with avocado frosting	40-41
raspberry jam & caramel semla	44-45
semla with chocolate and nuts	58-59
smulpaj	46-47
schackrutor	70-71
solar plexus crumb	87
strawberry gel	109

T

thermometer	25
turmeric powder	23
tiramisu	
tiramisu the Swedish way	84-85
tiramisu cake classic	116-117
truffle heliodor	86-87

V

vanilla bean powder	22
vacuum cleaner	48-49, 50, 51

Y

young coconut meat	19

RAW FIKA

about the author

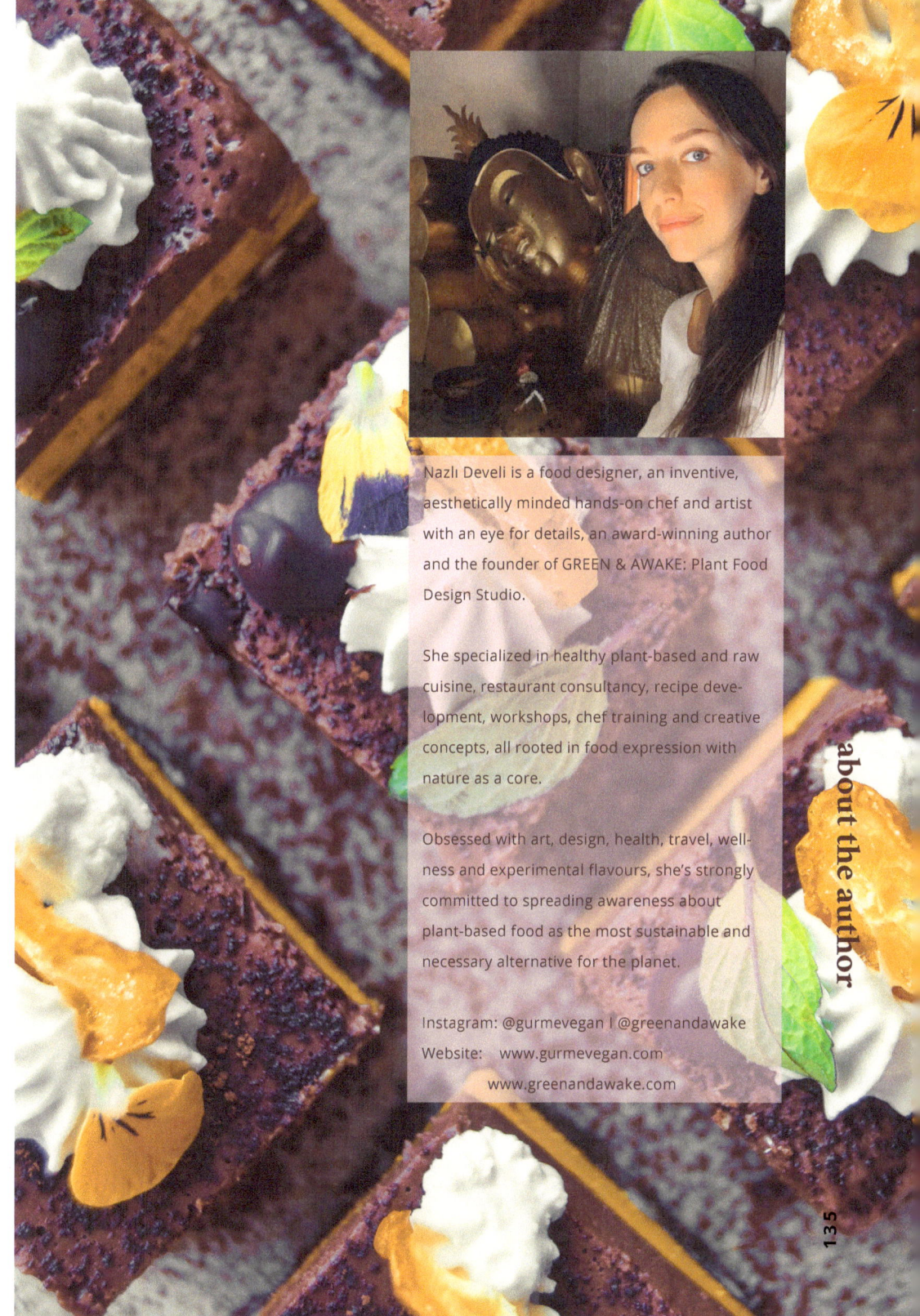

Nazlı Develi is a food designer, an inventive, aesthetically minded hands-on chef and artist with an eye for details, an award-winning author and the founder of GREEN & AWAKE: Plant Food Design Studio.

She specialized in healthy plant-based and raw cuisine, restaurant consultancy, recipe development, workshops, chef training and creative concepts, all rooted in food expression with nature as a core.

Obsessed with art, design, health, travel, wellness and experimental flavours, she's strongly committed to spreading awareness about plant-based food as the most sustainable and necessary alternative for the planet.

Instagram: @gurmevegan | @greenandawake
Website: www.gurmevegan.com
            www.greenandawake.com

www.ingramcontent.com/pod-product-compliance
Lightning Source LLC
Chambersburg PA
CBHW040722060526
44119CB00080B/297